Period Pain

Endometriosis, Fibroids, and the Fight for Better Women's Healthcare

SARAH CHITONGO

First published in the United Kingdom 2026.

A CIP catalogue record for this book is available from the British Library.

Printed and bound in Great Britain. PUR perfect-bound paperback.

Inner pages: Munken Premium Cream 90gsm. Cover: 300gsm with soft-touch matte lamination and spot UV.

This book contains accounts of medical care, including diagnostic delay, dismissal and bereavement. Reader discretion advised.

Cover design: in-house. Interior design: in-house. Illustrations: editorial production team.

Author's Note

A note, before we begin, about who I am and what you are about to read.

I am an NHS-trained nurse and midwife. I am a researcher. I hold a Queen's Nurse title and a Mary Seacole Award, one of the things I am proudest of in my professional life. I have taught midwifery at Middlesex University. I have presented my research at Downing Street and in Parliament, most of it concerning maternal health inequalities for Black, Asian and ethnic minority women in the United Kingdom. I am also the founder of Vina, a women's health platform that I built because the gaps I describe in these pages are real, and because someone needed to start filling them. I want you to know all of that up front, so that it cannot hang between us for the rest of the book.

I want you to know something else, too. I have not written this book as a memoir. I have made my own peace with my own body in rooms the reader does not need to enter, and I am not the story here. The women I have cared for, interviewed, and researched alongside are the story. It is my role to listen carefully to their voices in this book, to make sense of them in light of the best information available, and to state clearly what I have learned from 20 years of experience.

This book takes a position. It is written from a position that British medicine has been failing women in pain for generations, that the failure is architectural rather than accidental, and that the time for incremental change has passed. I will welcome the progress where there is progress. On 15 April 2026, the Department of Health and Social Care published the Renewed Women's Health Strategy for England, signed by the Secretary of State and with a foreword that names medical misogyny inside an NHS document for the first time (DHSC, 2026). That matters. I will cite it, draw on it, and hold the government to its commitments. But I will also ask the hard question of any strategy: whether the lived experience of women in the years to come resembles the promises on paper.

References are in Harvard style at the back of the book. Where I quote a woman by name from published reporting, I say so and cite the source. Where a story has been shared with me in confidence, names have been changed, and I flag that too. Nothing in this book is invented.

Finally, I will use the words "woman" and "women" throughout. I hold in mind that trans men, non-binary people and intersex people can experience endometriosis, fibroids and adenomyosis, and I do not wish to exclude anyone from the argument of this book. Where it matters for precision, I say "people who menstruate" or "people with uteruses". Most of the research I cite uses the language of women. I have tried to honour both the inclusive reality and the scientific record.

With that said, I am glad you are here.

Sarah Chitongo

London, April 2026

Contents

Preface

"The doctor listens, nods, types. And then she tells you: periods are like that for some women."

I have been in that room a thousand times.

I have been there as a midwife, standing beside the bed, observing a woman try to describe a pain that is beyond description and without witness. I have been there as a researcher, carrying questionnaires into NHS trusts and listening to what women say when they think, for once, that someone is actually asking. I have been there as a nurse, as a lecturer, as a policy voice in a Whitehall meeting where a statistic about Black maternal mortality was being discussed as though it were the weather. And I have sat, many times, across from a woman who came to me not because she had run out of doctors, but because she had run out of hope that a doctor would listen.

This book is for her.

It is also for the 1.5 million women in the UK who are currently living with endometriosis (Endometriosis UK, 2024). It is for the seven to eight women in every ten who will develop fibroids by the age of fifty, with 80% of Black women affected, compared to 70% of white women (Stewart et al., 2017; Scottish Government, 2026). It is for the women in the most detailed English survey we have ever done, the 2025 Reproductive Health Survey for England, who reported that nearly three-quarters of us are living with some form of poor reproductive health (Palmer et al., 2025). It is for the girl who is thirteen and already missing school because of a pain her mother has quietly taught her to bear. It is for the woman who is thirty-two and has just been told, for the ninth time, that periods are just like that for some women.

We have, as a country, built a system that does to women in pain exactly what it has done for generations. It reassures. It defers. It sends her home with a prescription for something mild and a note to come back if things do not improve. And then, when she comes back, and comes back, and comes back, it wonders aloud whether perhaps she is simply sensitive, or anxious, or unlucky with her cycles. The average wait for an endometriosis diagnosis in England is now nine years and four months (DHSC, 2026). This is what we have been calling care.

Nine years and four months. This is what we have been calling care.
And it has to stop.

In April of this year, the government published the Renewed Women's Health Strategy for England. Its opening sentences, signed by the Secretary of State for Health and Social Care, read: "The NHS has a problem with basic, everyday sexism and an appalling culture of medical misogyny" (DHSC, 2026, p. 2). A government department has named it. That matters. This book takes the Strategy seriously as both evidence and benchmark. It cites the commitments. And it asks, throughout, the question every woman reading this already has in her mind: how much of what is promised on paper will reach the waiting room she sits in next month.

I want to be honest with you about what this book is.

It is not a memoir. I have made my own peace with my own body in rooms the reader does not need to enter, and I am not the story here. The women I have cared for, interviewed, and researched alongside are the story. Women like Jen Moore, who spent twenty-two years being told her pain was ordinary before a surgeon finally opened her up and confirmed it was not. Women like Hayley, whose largest fibroid was the size of a mango, and who at twenty-six was asked by her doctor whether she really wanted to pursue a diagnosis because it would require surgery. Women like Sarah Beaton, who is alive today because she paid fifteen thousand pounds for a private scan that found uterine cancer, the NHS was going to make her wait eighteen months for (STV News, 2025). Women like Natalie, a Black British woman, were told by a GP that she could not have endometriosis because "it's what Black women get", meaning, in his mind, fibroids as though her ethnicity had pre-diagnosed her (Refinery29, 2025). Women like Lupita Nyong'o, who sat in front of an American television camera in February this year and said, of her fibroids, "nobody is helping. Nobody knows what to do to mitigate them" (TODAY, 2026).

These women are not anomalies. They are the pattern.

This book is also not a textbook, although it contains research, and I will not apologise for being careful with the evidence. What it is, above all, is a reckoning. A reckoning with a healthcare system that has normalised the pain of half its population for so long that women themselves have learned to call it ordinary. A reckoning with the idea that suffering is a tax on being a woman, and particularly on being a Black or Brown or poor or dismissed woman. A reckoning with the nine-minute consultation that was never going to be long enough to hear the truth of a body, and with the reassurance that was never going to be adequate in place of an investigation.

And it is a fight.

I have been fighting, in one form or another, for most of my professional life. I have taken my research into the House of Commons. I have sat in rooms at Number 10 Downing Street. I have learned, in every one of those rooms, that the women whose pain is the worst are not the women whose voices are the loudest. They are the women who have been taught, sometimes over generations, that complaining is weakness, that the body when it fails does so privately, and that the correct response to a pain a doctor cannot see is to get on with it. I do not believe that any more. I am not sure I ever did.

If you are reading this, I suspect you do not believe it either. Perhaps you have been reassured one too many times. Perhaps you have left a consultation in tears, you were careful not to cry until you were in the car, because crying in the room would have confirmed for the doctor what he was already saying out loud about your emotional state. Perhaps you have watched your mother do the same, and your sister do the same, and you have wondered how many of us there must be for this to keep happening and to keep being called normal.

There are, on the most conservative estimate, millions. In the United Kingdom alone. In our lifetimes. In this generation of women who were promised, with the founding of the NHS, a kind of care that would belong to them as a right. That care was never meant to be this.

You are not imagining it. You are not alone. And you are, finally, not unheard.

The book in your hands is, I hope, three things at once.

It is a validation. If you have been told you are making a fuss about nothing, you are not. The Endometriosis UK 2024 report, drawing on a survey of more than 4,300 diagnosed women, found that 78% had been told by at least one doctor they were "making a fuss about nothing", up from 69% in the same charity's 2020 survey (Endometriosis UK, 2024). You are not imagining it. You are not alone.

It is a map. Across these chapters, I will set out what endometriosis and fibroids actually are, how British medicine tends to fail at diagnosing them, where the treatment pathways work and where they break, and what the evidence says about how women can support their own bodies while they fight for the care they deserve. There are scripts in the back of this book for the next appointment. There is a checklist of symptoms that should never be reassured away. There is a directory of the specialist centres you have the right to be referred to. That's what these pages were intended for: They were supposed to be dog-eared, photographed, and sent in WhatsApp group chats.

Because this struggle will not become any easier until women are no longer burdened by it alone. The Royal Colleges know that. The Members of Parliament know that. The commissioners know that. It's been in the data on their desks for decades now. What has been missing is not information. What has been missing is the will.

The time for this book is now because the gynaecology waiting list in England is 565,000 women long (NHS England, 2026). It is now because Lupita Nyong'o is on American television, saying nobody is helping. It is now because MPs debated this on the floor of the House of Commons in March of this year and used the phrase "shameful delays" (Hansard, 2026). It is now because the Renewed Women's Health Strategy has, for the first time, written medical misogyny into a government document and because what happens next depends on whether women refuse to let that commitment dissolve into the usual delay.

We are at an inflexion point. Books like this one are part of how a country turns.

I have written the one I wished existed when I began. I hope, before you put it down, that you will have underlined something, written to your MP, shared the Patient Manifesto at the back of the book, used the script with your GP, or simply sat quietly for a moment and let yourself believe that what has been happening to you is not your fault, and was never yours to carry alone.

Then I hope you will join me.

The fight is long and old. From here on in, it is not a fight any of us will lose alone.

SC

PART I

Living with Period Pain

CHAPTER ONE

What Period Pain Really Looks Like

Aaliyah is fourteen years old, and she has missed eleven days of school in the last term.

Her mother brought her to see me not as a clinician in that moment, but as a family friend because she did not know where else to turn. The GP had said Aaliyah's periods were heavy but within the range of normal for a girl her age. A nurse had suggested she try a warmer hot water bottle and perhaps paracetamol taken more regularly. Her mother had tried everything she could remember her own mother trying, and none of it was working. Aaliyah was pale from blood loss. She was doubling over in the evenings and crying in a way that her mother said she had not cried since she was small. On two occasions that term, she had had to leave a lesson because the blood had gone through a super-tampon, a pad and her uniform trousers within an hour.

She sat on the edge of my sofa and asked me, without looking up, whether this was going to be her whole life now.
That question is the reason for this book.

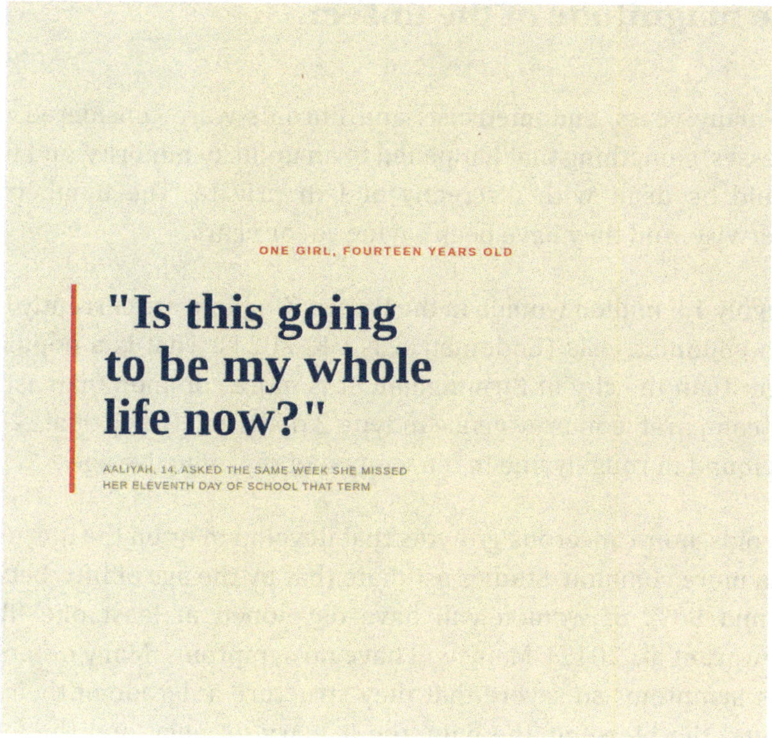

Figure 1. Aaliyah, fourteen.

This chapter is about what period pain actually looks like in Britain in 2026, not in the abstracts of a textbook, but in the lives of the women and girls whose bodies do not behave the way they have been told bodies behave. We will look at the scale of what is happening in our country. We will meet some of the women whose names and stories thread through every chapter of this book. And we will begin to trace, together, the shape of the system that has been failing them.

I need you to understand that if you're reading this in the kitchen late at night, commuting on your way home, or sitting in a waiting room after having been there for two hours, that this suffering that you bear is not minor, or common, or your fault. Nor is it, according to any objective interpretation of the facts, uncommon.

The magnitude of the unseen

For many years, endometriosis and fibroids were considered niche illnesses, something that happened to an unlucky minority, and which should be dealt with discreetly and in private. The numbers say otherwise, and they have been saying so for years.

Roughly 1.5 million women in the United Kingdom are currently living with endometriosis (Endometriosis UK, 2024). That is a population larger than the city of Birmingham. It is more common than asthma, and comparable in prevalence to type 2 diabetes (Okoth et al., 2021). It is found in roughly one in ten women of reproductive age.

Fibroids, non-cancerous growths that develop in or on the uterus, are even more common. Studies estimate that by the age of fifty, between 70 and 80% of women will have developed at least one fibroid (Stewart et al., 2017). Many will have no symptoms. Many others will have symptoms so severe that they structure a decade of their lives around the bleeding, the pain, the urinary urgency, and the fatigue that iron deficiency brings. Research consistently shows that Black women are disproportionately affected: approximately 80% will develop fibroids by age fifty, compared to 70% of white women, and they tend to develop them earlier, in greater numbers, and with more severe symptoms (Scottish Government, 2026; Stewart et al., 2017; Katon et al., 2023).

Adenomyosis, a condition in which endometrial tissue grows into the muscular wall of the uterus, is less well studied in the UK and still frequently missed on imaging. It is often discussed alongside endometriosis, and in practice, they overlap often enough that many women live with both, a fact that sometimes takes years to establish even after a first diagnosis.

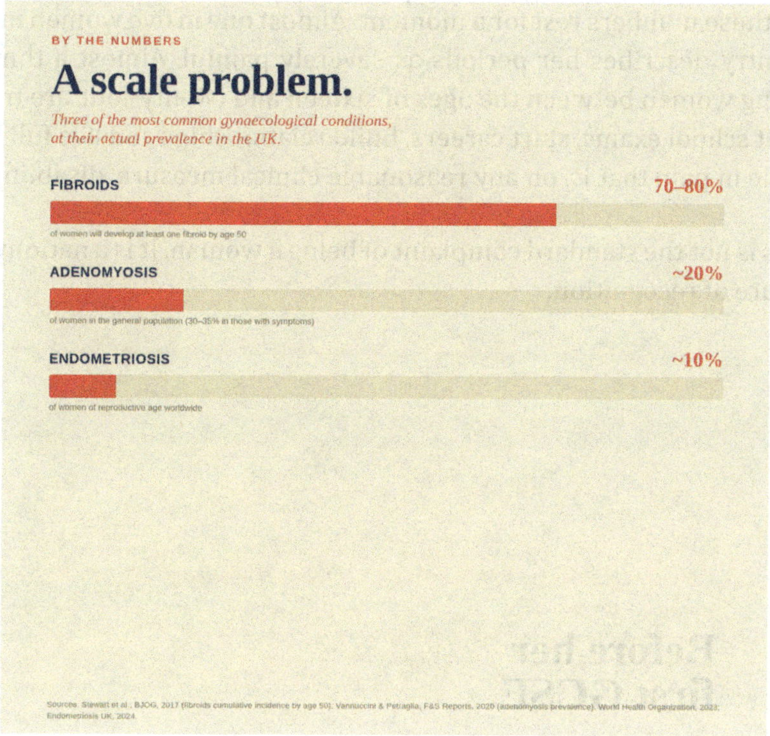

Figure 2. Prevalence: fibroids, adenomyosis, endometriosis.

In November 2025, the British Journal of Obstetrics and Gynaecology published the results of the Reproductive Health Survey for England, the largest study of its kind ever conducted in this country. Nearly 60,000 women and people assigned female at birth took part. Among the findings: 73.7% of respondents reported at least one measure of poor reproductive health in the preceding year (Palmer et al., 2025). Almost three in four. Menstrual-related problems were reported by 61.9%. Severely painful periods were reported by 18.7% of all women, and among women aged 16 to 24, that figure rose to above 30% (Palmer et al., 2025).

Let those numbers rest for a moment. Almost one in five women in this country describes her periods as severely painful. Almost a third of young women between the ages of sixteen and twenty-four are trying to sit school exams, start careers, build relationships and live full lives while in pain that is, on any reasonable clinical measure, disabling.

This is not the standard complaint of being a woman. It is a nationwide failure of recognition.

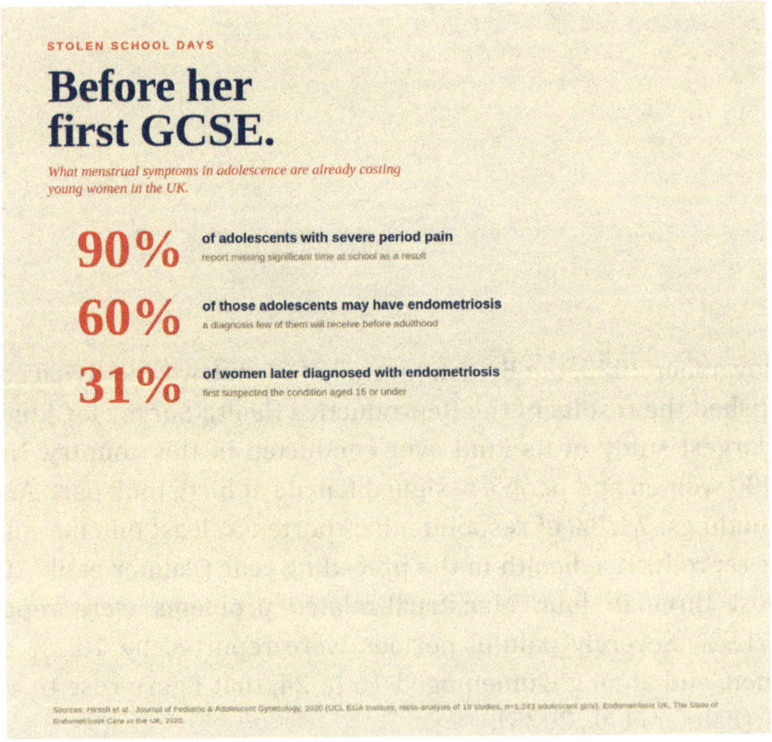

Figure 3. Stolen school days.

Beyond the pelvis

One of the most persistent misconceptions about endometriosis is that it is a disease of the uterus. It is not. Endometriosis is a whole-body condition. Tissue similar to the endometrial lining grows in places it should not: on the ovaries, on the bowel, on the bladder, on the diaphragm, in rare cases in the lungs, the eye, and even on the brain (Chapron et al., 2019). Because this tissue responds to the hormonal cycle, it bleeds each month. Unlike the endometrial lining, it has nowhere to go. The result is inflammation, adhesions, scarring, cysts, and pain that can radiate into parts of the body a woman may never think to connect to her periods.

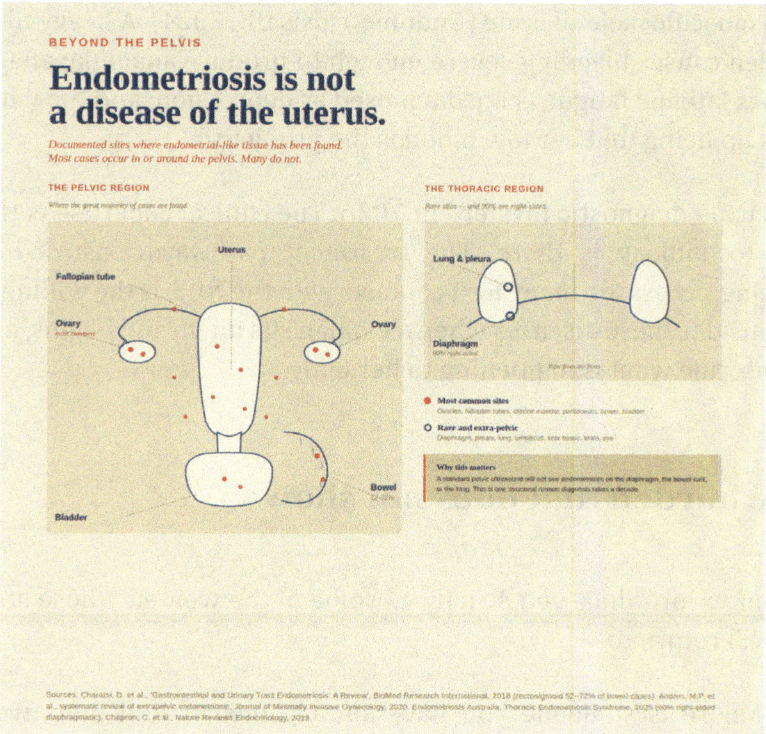

Figure 4. Endometriosis is not a disease of the uterus.

Jen Moore, whose story will return across this book, describes endometriosis as having "been discovered to exist in all organs of the human body, including the eye, the bone, and the belly button" (Moore, cited in Endometriosis UK, 2024). She is right. And she spent twenty-two years explaining to GPs, gynaecologists, and A&E doctors that the pain she was describing in her shoulder, her chest, her bowel was connected to her cycle, before she finally met a surgeon who believed her enough to look.

Fibroids present differently, but with a similarly wide reach. A large fibroid pressing on the bladder produces constant urinary urgency. One pressing on the bowel produces constipation that no amount of fibre will fix. A fibroid against the spine as in the case of Hayley, a British woman whose mango-sized tumour was only discovered in her early thirties produces back pain that can be mistaken for years for a musculoskeletal issue (Endometriosis UK, 2024). A heavy fibroid burden causes bleeding severe enough to produce anaemia; anaemia causes fatigue; fatigue is misdiagnosed as depression; and the woman ends up being told her low mood is the problem.

This is no diagnostic mystery in 2026. The clinical expertise is there. The technology is there. The treatment pathways exist. What is missing, across too many first contacts with the NHS, is the willingness to consider these diseases when a woman sits down and begins, again, to describe what is happening to her body.

The burden that does not show

I want to introduce you, briefly, to some of the women whose stories we will return to.

Jen Moore is someone you have already met. It took her twenty-two years from first experiencing excruciating pain to receiving her diagnosis. She speaks out for herself now, having done more to inform public opinion in Britain about endometriosis than any press statement released by the Department of Health ever did.

Hayley was thirty-two when an abdominal ultrasound, ordered as part of a cancer scare, found four large fibroids, including the mango pressed against her spine (Endometriosis UK, 2024). She had been in pain since adolescence. At twenty-six, a doctor raised the possibility of endometriosis but then asked her, in a tone of shared reasonableness, whether she really wanted to pursue a diagnosis given that it would require surgery. She said no. When the fibroids were finally discovered, her first reaction was not fear, but relief: the pain was real. She had not imagined it. She was not too sensitive, too anxious, or too focused on her health. We will return to Hayley's relief, because it is the most damning line in this book.

Sarah Beaton, forty-three, from Elgin in Scotland, was referred to her local NHS hospital after months of painful periods. An initial scan revealed a fibroid. She was told she faced an eighteen-month wait for treatment. Because she was worried, in her words, "just worried", she paid £15,000 in January 2025 for a private scan at Aberdeen's Albyn Hospital (STV News, 2025). Two weeks later, she had a full hysterectomy. The scan had found cancer in her uterus. "If I'd waited, I'd be none the wiser," she said. Later, she added a line I keep coming back to: "In effect, people are dying on the waiting lists because they're not getting the treatment they need when they need it." Sarah Beaton is alive because she had fifteen thousand pounds. Hold that fact.

Natalie is thirty-three. She is Black British. She was finally diagnosed with endometriosis at thirty-three, after thirteen years of trying. Years earlier, a GP had told her she could not have endometriosis because "it's what Black women get", meaning fibroids, which the doctor had assumed on sight. Natalie told him her white mother had endometriosis. He still did not believe her (Refinery29, 2025). She has since had five surgeries. She was also, at a late stage, told she was no longer eligible for NHS fertility treatment. We will return to Natalie's consultation room in Chapter Four, and we will return to her loss of eligibility in Chapter Seven.

Leanne Pickering spent twelve years in pain before she was diagnosed with endometriosis. She then faced a two-year NHS wait for surgery and spent £10,000 on private care (BBC News, 2025). "They won't let me see my endometriosis specialist if I don't do this checklist," she told reporters, describing a system that required her to repeat investigations she had already had. She had been diagnosed. She knew what she needed. The system still insisted on its own process.

And finally, because this is a global story as well as a British one, Lupita Nyong'o. In February 2026, the Academy Award winning actress sat on the TODAY show and spoke plainly about her fibroids. In 2014, the year of her Oscar win, she had surgery to remove the fibroids she was carrying. Twelve years later, she has more than 50, the largest the size of an orange. In her own words, on her 43rd birthday in March 2026: "Over the course of my lifetime, I have carried 77 uterine fibroids: 25 surgically removed and more than 50 still growing inside me today." "I was so upset because I feel powerless," she told the programme. "It's a ticking bomb. They're going haywire in my body, and nobody is helping. Nobody knows what to do to mitigate them" (TODAY, 2026). She has since partnered with the Foundation for Women's Health to launch a fibroid research fund and is co-sponsoring the US U-FIGHT Act, seeking $150 million in research funding over five years (Complex, 2026).

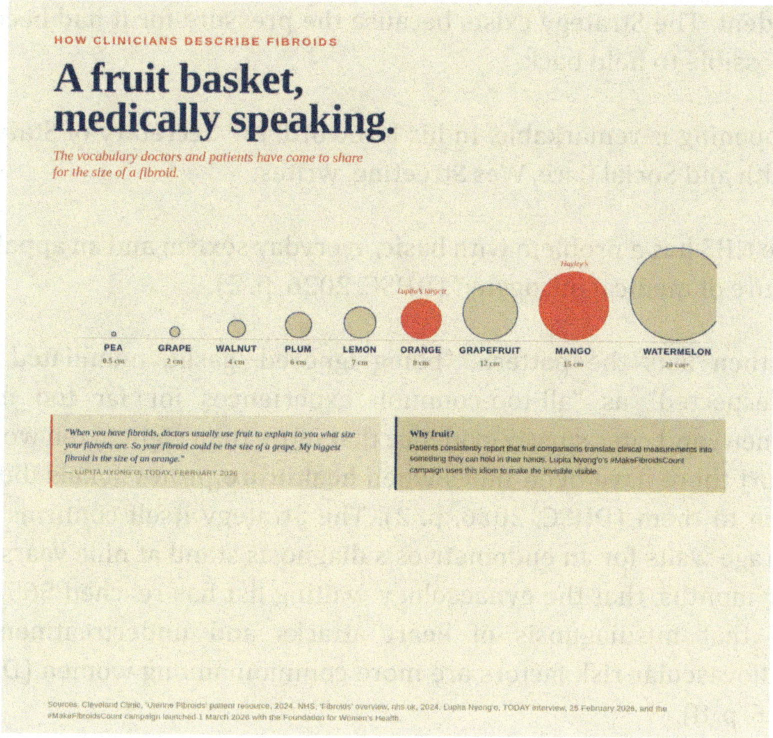

Figure 5. A fruit basket, medically speaking.

Six women. Six lives. The oldest sixty, the youngest fourteen. Between them, more than a century of explaining a pain nobody wanted to investigate.

And these are the ones whose names we know.

What the system now admits

This book was finished in the spring of 2026, which happens to be the same moment the Department of Health and Social Care published its Renewed Women's Health Strategy for England. The timing is not an accident. The Strategy exists because the pressure for it had become impossible to hold back.

Its opening is remarkable. In his foreword, the Secretary of State for Health and Social Care, Wes Streeting, writes:

"The NHS has a problem with basic, everyday sexism and an appalling culture of medical misogyny" (DHSC, 2026, p. 2).

He then lists the pattern: "being ignored, gaslit, humiliated and disrespected" as "all-too-common experiences for far too many women", and cites survey evidence that more than eight in ten women report there have been times when healthcare professionals did not listen to them (DHSC, 2026, p. 2). The Strategy itself confirms that average waits for an endometriosis diagnosis stand at nine years and four months, that the gynaecology waiting list has reached 565,000, and that misdiagnosis of heart attacks and undertreatment of cardiovascular risk factors are more common among women (DHSC, 2026, p. 8).

These are not activist claims any more. They are the government's own position.

Something has shifted. I want to be careful, though, because I have seen strategies before. The 2022 Women's Health Strategy under the previous government made many of the same observations; the Renewed Strategy is itself explicit that its predecessor "was set up to fail because it operated within and accepted an outmoded care model" (DHSC, 2026, p. 9). A strategy is only worth its implementation. This book is an argument for holding the current one to the fire of actual delivery, not for taking its promises as completed work.

But the acknowledgement matters. A woman who has been told for twenty years that her pain is within the range of normal for women can now hand the Secretary of State's own words back to her GP and say: He doesn't think so.

What period pain actually looks like

So, what does it actually look like?

It looks like a fourteen-year-old missing three weeks of school each term and being told that her periods are within the normal range.

It looks like a twenty-six-year-old paying for a private ultrasound because her GP will not refer her.

It looks like a thirty-three-year-old fighting for thirteen years to be told she has a condition her doctor told her she could not have because of the colour of her skin.

It looks like a forty-three-year-old spending £15,000 to find a cancer that the NHS was going to let her wait eighteen months for.

It looks like 565,000 women in England are currently on a gynaecology waiting list, 57% of whom have been waiting less than eighteen weeks, meaning 43% have been waiting longer than the NHS's own target (NHS England, 2026). It looks like more than a quarter of those on the waiting list have already been to Accident and Emergency because of their condition, more than one in ten of those requiring emergency intervention such as blood transfusion (RCOG, 2026).

It looks like being told that your pain is ordinary. And then waking up, still in it.

It looks like a quiet, not polite, but exhausted refusal to believe that this is the care our country is capable of providing to half its population.

This book is written on the basis that refusal is growing.

The next chapter is about how the refusal most often starts: in a room, with a stranger, who has been trained to reassure rather than investigate. That mechanism has a name. I am going to give it one, and then we are going to dismantle it.

※ ※ ※

CHAPTER TWO

The Reassurance Trap

Sarah Beaton is forty-three, and she is alive because she did not trust the NHS.

In January 2025, a scan at Aberdeen's Albyn Hospital, which she paid £15,000 for, found cancer in her uterus. Two weeks later, she had a full hysterectomy. Had she stayed on the NHS waiting list, her GP had placed her on after finding what was then thought to be a routine fibroid, she would have waited another eighteen months. By then, she told STV News in a short, flat sentence I cannot stop thinking about, "I'd be none the wiser" (STV News, 2025).

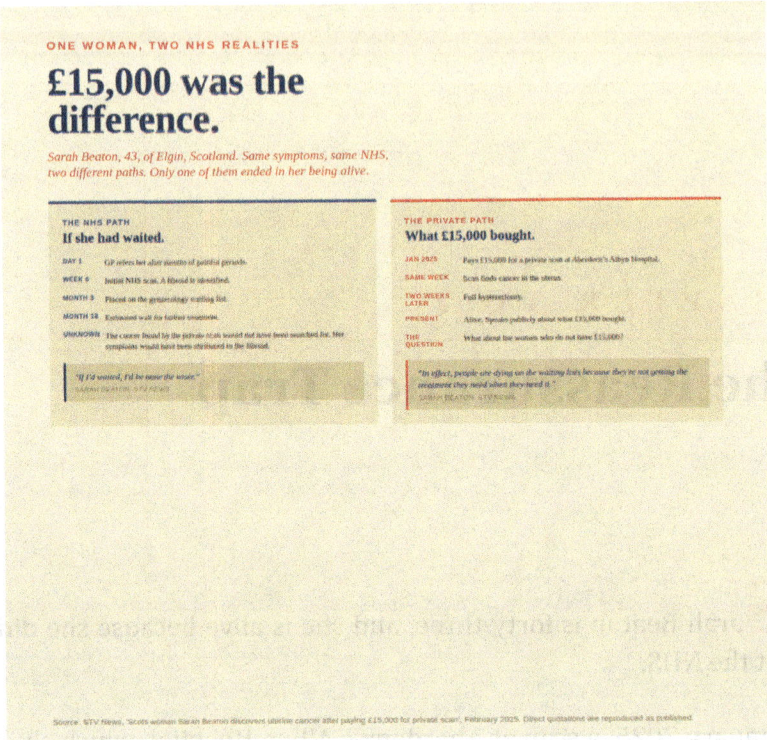

Figure 6. £15,000 was the difference. Sarah Beaton's two paths.

Sit with that for a moment. It is the sound of a woman discovering that she very nearly died in a queue.

I am beginning with Sarah because her story does something statistics cannot. It collapses the distance between an abstraction and a life. This chapter is, on one level, about abstractions: the nine years and four months it takes on average to receive an endometriosis diagnosis in the UK (DHSC, 2026); the 565,000 women currently on the gynaecology waiting list in England (NHS England, 2026); the 78% of women eventually diagnosed with endometriosis who remember being told, by at least one doctor, that they were making a fuss about nothing (Endometriosis UK, 2024). These are astonishing numbers.

They are also, by design, easy to skim past. A statistic is a life with its edges filed off.

Sarah's edges are sharp. So are Jen's, whom we will come back to in a moment, and Hayley's, and Natalie's, and Lupita's, and all the women in this book, and the millions more whose names I will never learn. What they share is not their diagnosis. Endometriosis and fibroids are different conditions with different biologies and different treatments.

This common thread is an experience they've all had before, alongside, and instead of a diagnosis. This has no NHS code. This has no medical name. This lies unspoken in every consultation where a woman is told her pain is normal, and she goes home.

I will call this the reassurance trap.

By naming it, I have come to realise that we begin to break free from it.

Shape of the trap

This is how it happens.

A lady turns up at her doctor's office with symptoms of pain. The pain is real. The pain is cyclical; it is tied to her period, around the time of ovulation, or it has become a tag-along between periods, like a pesky stalker who refuses to give up. She did not arrive there lightly. In nearly all scenarios, she would have tried over-the-counter pain relief pills, the hot water bottle, what her mother said, what her sister recommended, something she read on social media, or maybe just the tiny doubt in her mind saying, "Surely it can't be that bad."

Doctors are nice people. Most doctors are. Doctors have nine minutes. Most doctors have, according to Irving et al., the average appointment with a general practitioner in the United Kingdom lasts 9.2 minutes

(2017). The Renewed Women's Health Strategy itself recognises that the structure of the consultation imposes limitations on what happens during it (DHSC, 2026). Doctors do not know who she is, and have not had the opportunity to review the eight previous consultations listed on the computer screen. In nine minutes, with someone she does not know, through the half partition of conversation, the doctor says something like: "Some women experience their periods like that." Or: "Have you tried taking a different Pill?" Or: "Let's see if it settles."

The woman takes her script, or doesn't, and a little flash of relief goes with her. The doctor has said that she is fine. She wishes to believe him. She will try.

Within her, whatever it may be, the sickness persists.

This is the trap. It is constructed from well-meaning motives, limited resources, and the hard mathematical fact that most women entering their office with period pains are not suffering from either endometriosis or fibroids. They are suffering from poor periods, and in this context, the physician's optimistic response is, mathematically speaking, correct. This is why the trap can hold its shape so effectively. It closes again and again on the women for whom optimism is precisely the wrong solution, and it is endlessly justified as common sense by all those whose fault it is.

Jen Moore spent twenty-two years breaking out of it.

Jen

Jen Moore is currently an activist for endometriosis sufferers. She is on the radio. She has conversations with Members of Parliament. Jen is the face that is always cited by the major press releases on the topic in Britain, and anyone familiar with the online community for endometriosis patients is sure to recognise the voice. Sharp, frustrated, and with humour that comes only from years and years of experience.

Twenty-two years. At thirteen, the pain began; at thirty-five, it became clear that someone would have to open her up and verify for her what her body had been trying to tell her all of her adult life.

Between those two dates is a life, and the things in life that cannot be done due to pain. Exam periods spent in a state of fugue. Illnesses treated with such scarcity as wartime sugar. Love affairs where eventually one must confess that sometimes she does not feel well enough to have sex, that sometimes it is not simply a matter of moods or evasions or lack of understanding on her part when she says she just does not know why. Workplaces where even her bosses see the pattern first. The suspicion shifts from the outside world to herself. Perhaps I am exaggerating. Perhaps other women know this and just deal.

As Jen states, "The problem is that we do not believe women." I will take it even one step further and say that we train women not to believe themselves.

The numbers, briefly

I promised statistics, and I will keep the promise, because the scale of this is part of the story. I will then put them down and go back to the women.

Endometriosis UK's 2024 survey of more than 4,300 diagnosed women remains the best picture we have of the British diagnostic journey. The average wait from first symptoms to confirmed diagnosis is eight years and ten months in England and Scotland, nine years and five months in Northern Ireland, and nine years and eleven months in Wales (Endometriosis UK, 2024). The government's own Renewed Women's Health Strategy now quotes a figure of nine years and four months as the UK average (DHSC, 2026). A decade, functionally, for a woman in Cardiff to get an answer.

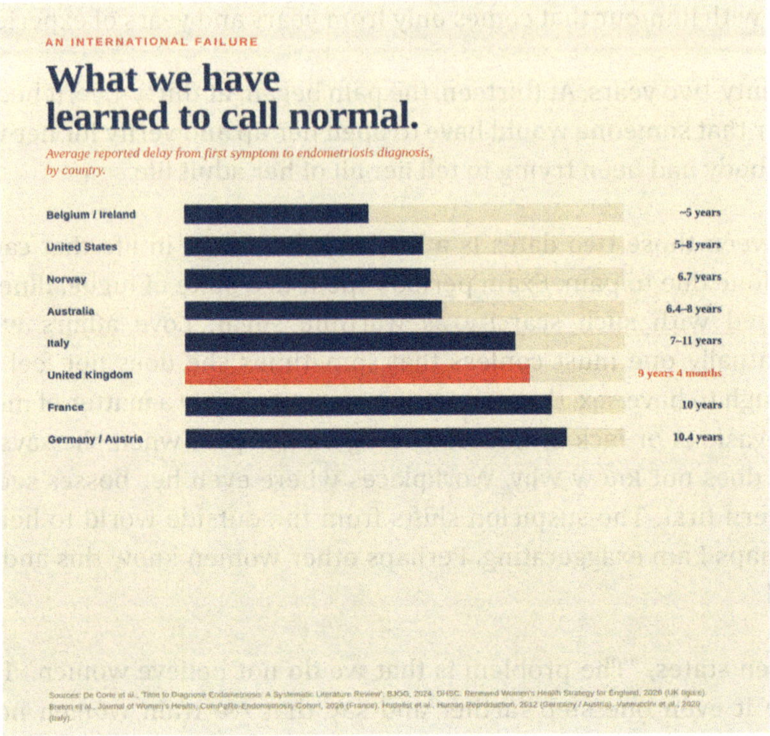

Figure 7. Average diagnostic delay for endometriosis, by country.

47% of women go to their GP ten or more times before diagnosis. 70% go at least five. 52% have been to A&E with their symptoms. A quarter has been three or more times. Fewer than one in five of those A&E visits result in a gynaecology referral (Endometriosis UK, 2024).

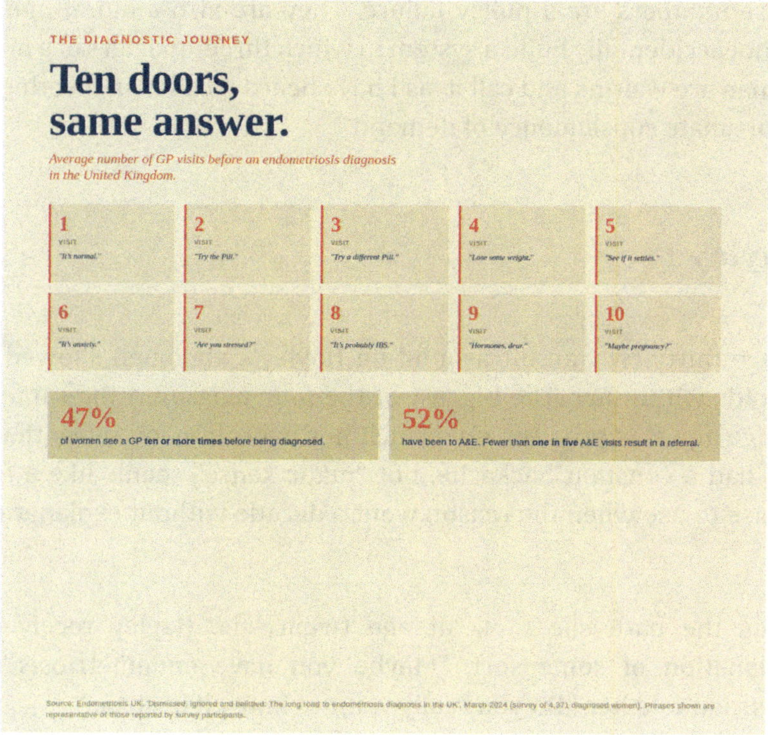

Figure 8. Ten doors, same answer.

Now, the delay after diagnosis, because the delay does not stop once someone has finally said the word. As of January 2026, 565,000 women were on the gynaecology waiting list in England (NHS England, 2026). The Royal College of Obstetricians and Gynaecologists reports that 43% of them had been waiting longer than the 18-week target (RCOG, 2026). In Scotland, nearly 13,000 women are currently waiting, and 324 of them have been waiting more than three years (McKirdy, 2025). Three years is the length of a degree. Three years is a school age. Three years is a very long time to be in pain and know that someone, somewhere, has a spreadsheet with your name on it and is not, today, going to call.

These numbers are a policy failure. They are also a moral one. You cannot accidentally build a system in which three-quarters of a million women are waiting and call it, as I have heard it called in meetings, an unfortunate consequence of demand.

Hayley

At age thirty-two, an ultrasound on Hayley's abdomen showed four fibroids within her. The biggest of the four measured the same as a mango and was pressing up against her back. It made sense that she had had a constant backache, but "made sense" seems like a funny phrase to use when the reason went a decade without explanation to her.

Along the path she took, at age twenty-six, Hayley received an explanation of some sort. "Maybe you have endometriosis," one physician told her. "Do you really want to know if it's true?"

Consider how that question is constructed. It seems sensible. It seems patient-centred. It seems, indeed, like shared decision making, which is what everyone is supposed to be striving for from their doctors nowadays. Consider it from another angle. In asking this question, the responsibility of "shall we look into this?" rests upon a young woman, aged twenty-six, who has been living a life full of misery caused by years of pain. Uncertainty is cast as the safer choice, while finding out is considered a riskier option.

Hayley, predictably, declined. "Who would?" she noted later. By this point, rumours were being whispered about how maybe she was too concerned about her health, too nervous. She was already beginning to accept what women in her situation invariably do: to agree with them. The reason for her failure to be diagnosed was due to her growing rational doubt regarding her body's own account (Endometriosis UK, 2024).

This is the truest cruelty of the trap: making the woman believe herself a liar before citing her refusal to speak as proof that all was fine.

What the trap is not

Before I continue, I must be cautious, for the last thing that a woman reading this wants is yet another tale of villainy. The reassurance trap is not the product of bad doctors. I have spoken to and read the testimony of GPs who work twelve-hour shifts in English primary care and carry genuine, career-long grief about the women they failed to refer. The system is designed in a way that causes their failure and then blames them for it.

A nine-minute consultation is not a clinical encounter. It is a bureaucratic unit. Inside it, a GP is expected to take a history, conduct any necessary examination, arrive at a differential, write a prescription, document everything, and decide whether to spend one of their rationed referrals on this patient or the next one in the corridor. The structural default reassures, ask her to come back if it gets worse, defer the decision to a later appointment is not laziness. It is what a nine-minute unit is built to produce.

The Renewed Women's Health Strategy is, to its credit, honest about this. It describes the NHS care model as "one size fits all", "too focused on provider interests, rather than patient interests", and "highly paternalistic, centralised and bureaucratic" (DHSC, 2026, p. 9). It acknowledges, in effect, that the architecture is the problem.

The trap, in other words, is architectural. It is not caused by individual dismissal, though individual dismissal lives inside it and is often what the woman remembers. It is caused by the shape of the room. Which is why fixing it requires more than telling GPs to listen harder.

Gaslight, dismissed, hysteria.

Still, shape-of-the-room explanations only take us so far, because the room also runs on a set of beliefs about women's pain that predate nine-minute appointments by a couple of thousand years.

Medical gaslighting, the pattern by which patients are made to doubt their own experiences of their bodies, is now a phrase in wide circulation. It appears in the medical literature, in patient advocacy, and, as of 2025, in the Women and Equalities Committee's inquiry into women's reproductive health conditions (Women and Equalities Committee, 2024). Dr Beth Malory, a health communication researcher at University College London, has written persuasively about what she calls the privileging of the "medical gaze", the bias baked into clinical training towards what can be seen, measured, imaged, and therefore believed (Malory, 2023). Endometriosis, notoriously, cannot be confirmed on a standard ultrasound. Fibroids can be, but only if someone orders the scan. In the gap between symptom and scan, in the territory where the only evidence is the woman's own testimony, British medicine has a long and unattractive history of deciding that testimony is not enough.

The gender pain gap is not an opinion. A 2024 survey commissioned by Nurofen found that 81% of women aged 18 to 24 reported having their pain dismissed or ignored by a healthcare professional, with 62% of all women reporting the same, a 27% rise since the previous year (Nurofen, 2024). A 2024 study in the Proceedings of the National Academy of Sciences found a systematic disparity in pain treatment for 21,000 patients attending emergency departments in the USA and Israel, with women significantly less likely than men to receive pain relief for equivalent complaints (Guzikevits et al., 2024). A British Journal of Pain study of UK Biobank participants found that chronic pain disproportionately affects women, and that women report more severe and impactful pain than men (Luo et al., 2026).

The Renewed Women's Health Strategy itself cites all three of these data points (DHSC, 2026, pp. 18–19). It acknowledges, quoting the 2022 call for evidence, that 84% of women reported times they were not listened to by healthcare professionals (DHSC, 2026, p. 18). One in three women reported severe pain scores of 7 or more out of 10 during NHS outpatient hysteroscopy procedures without sedation (RCOG, 2024, cited in DHSC, 2026, p. 22).

Eighty-four percent think about the ordinary statistical distribution of that figure for a moment. It means that if you are in a room with ten women, the chances are that only one or two of them have not, at some point, had a healthcare professional fail to listen to them.

I do not know of many indictments of a public service more total than that.

The cost of the wait

Let me return to the women. I keep returning to them because they are the point.

While a woman is caught in the trap, her condition does not pause. Every month, there is bleeding and scar tissue formation. The adhesions begin to grow. The fibroids get bigger. For many women, fertility may be compromised slowly and quietly, without fanfare, without any warning. According to an ONS report in 2025, women were earning less each month and were much less likely to be working than five years previously since their diagnosis, after adjusting for their age, number of births, and general economic activity (ONS, 2025).

The emotional toll is more difficult to measure than the economic. Each woman I have ever met or spoken to has her own take on what Hayley went through, the insidious process, the relative who delicately hints that perhaps she might be overthinking it, the point at which she starts believing them. That is where the viciousness of the cycle truly lies; it never ends with the diagnosis. The woman who has been convinced for ten years that her body cannot be trusted does not suddenly stop questioning herself once the expert validates her fears.

This particular grief seems to have its own unique pain that I feel like we don't discuss enough. When Hayley speaks of her reaction to the ultrasound, she does not speak of fear but of relief. Her pain was very real, and it had not been a dream. No one should need to be thankful for having a tumour the size of a mango compressing their spinal cord.

Two exits

What I'd like to conclude with is something practical, because criticism without an exit route can be a little cruel in itself.

There are two escape routes from the reassurance loop: one personal and one structural, and both are crucial.

The personal escape route, which women have been inventing for themselves for years now, and which is codified in this book in Appendix A, is basically a protocol. Write your dates and pain numbers and work, and sex and sleep disruptions down before the appointment. Take the paper in. In the appointment, ask one question that can't be avoided by the nine-minute format. The question is:

"What else might this be, and what tests would prove that?"

That does not come across as aggressive. It is clinical. The discussion is shifting from one of reassurance to differential diagnosis, which is the terminology that GPs work well with. The answer may still be that it's "wait and see," in which case the next line is:

"Would you please make a note in my record that I have asked for tests and been discouraged from doing so?"

This sentence, I am told by GPs whose judgement I trust, changes the room. It converts an informal encounter into a documented one, and documentation is a thing the NHS takes seriously in a way it has historically not taken women seriously.

The structural exit is larger, and it is not the patient's job. It involves mandatory gynaecology teaching in GP training, protected appointment time for suspected chronic gynaecological conditions, and the NICE guideline on endometriosis, which already exists, and recommends specialist referral after three months of persistent symptoms (NICE, 2017, updated 2024), actually being followed. The Renewed Women's Health Strategy makes several commitments in this direction. Action 28 promises a single point of access for gynaecology referrals within three years. Actions 4 and 5 commit to patient power payments in gynaecology and to a quality improvement programme using GP Patient Survey data to reduce variation in how GPs listen to women (DHSC, 2026, pp. 20–21). Jess's Rule, introduced in 2025 and named for a woman whose cancer was missed after more than twenty GP visits, now requires GP teams to "reflect, review, and rethink" if a patient presents three times with the same or worsening symptoms (DHSC, 2026, p. 2).

These are real commitments. Whether they reach Aaliyah's GP by the time Aaliyah is fifteen remains to be seen. That is the subject of the rest of this book.

Sarah Beaton paid £15,000 for the scan that found her cancer. I keep thinking about the women who cannot. I keep thinking about what kind of country has decided that a woman's chance of being diagnosed before a tumour becomes malignant is a question of her bank balance.

I keep thinking, too, about the thirteen-year-old Jen Moore, whose first bad period was in 1995 and whose diagnosis came in 2017, and about how much of her life was spent believing what she had been told. That this is what being a woman felt like, and she had better learn to bear it. She was not, it turned out, being dramatic.

Neither are you.

PART II

Navigating Care

CHAPTER THREE

Appointments, Pathways, and Gaps

Neelam Heera-Shergill is the founder of Cysters, a Birmingham charity that began in her living room and now supports women across the UK whose reproductive health has been failed by the system. Speaking to the Royal College of Obstetricians and Gynaecologists, she has been one of the clearest voices on the way the gynaecology waiting list lands harder on some women than others: "It is clear from the data what we have known all along. When there is an existing problem of women not being able to access gynaecological services promptly, health inequalities result in South Asian and black women being disadvantaged even more" (Heera-Shergill, quoted in RCOG, 2026).

Keep this in mind as you read on through the next few pages. The waiting list isn't a simple figure it's a distribution with its own distribution.

This chapter concerns itself with how the system really works when a woman attempts to get around it. We're going to examine the primary-care gatekeeper who decides to refer her. We'll consider specialist services and see if she can access them. We're going to see what the postcode lottery throws up. But mostly, we're asking ourselves, as this book is concerned with improving care rather than simply documenting failure, how the Renewed Women's Health Strategy's promises hold the key to getting out.

The gatekeeper

For virtually all women suffering from either endometriosis or fibroids, the patient's journey will invariably start with their GP. In many ways, the GP is the gatekeeper to the entire medical system. The GP is the very first person that a woman sees when she experiences pain or discomfort and will ultimately determine if further investigation is required or if she should be referred to a specialist.

And this issue is no small thing to consider in terms of structure. The GP has too much to bear; there are scores of people coming through his door daily with their own issues, chronic diseases that appear to have similarities, and a system that has to be rationed for referrals. When a woman walks into his office complaining of pain, bleeding, and tiredness, this is not an easy diagnosis. In the face of all this, the easiest way out is soothing and simply prescribing ibuprofen, and he will follow up in six weeks.

But the implications of this filtering role, even with the best of intentions, are truly devastating to those individuals whose symptoms deviate from the norm. The research carried out by Endometriosis UK indicated that almost fifty% of women suffering from endometriosis had to make at least ten visits to their GP before being formally diagnosed with the condition (Endometriosis UK, 2024). Ten visits, ten visits which involve time off from work, ten visits in which the patient must explain her symptoms, only to be told that it is "normal."

The issue is not only that GPs do not recognise these conditions, but the primary care system itself that makes such a task virtually impossible. Continuity of care is uncommon; women consult with new GPs every time, which starts the diagnostic process anew. The need to deal with demand implies that a referral to a specialist is made after much consideration, and numerous rounds of conservative treatment are pursued first by most GPs.

Women in marginalised populations are faced with additional obstacles when trying to access secondary care. According to the RCOG analysis, the number of patients on the waiting list increased most for Black and Asian women, and there is reason to believe that the number is understated due to the incompleteness of information about their ethnicity (RCOG, 2026). Women who live in the most disadvantaged areas represent the largest proportion of patients in prolonged wait times; 15% of patients who waited more than 52 weeks came from the most disadvantaged regions, while only 7% did from the least disadvantaged (RCOG, 2026).

The referral for those who survive many GP appointments is a sign of progression. However, the process does not represent progression from confusion to certainty. On the contrary, this is a progression from one broken step in healthcare to the next, and it is only the beginning of the waiting game.

The waiting rooms

Once referred to gynaecology, women enter a new phase of the journey: the waiting list. And here, the numbers are staggering.

As of January 2026, 565,000 women were on the gynaecology waiting list in England (NHS England, 2026). If every woman currently waiting stood shoulder to shoulder, the queue would stretch for miles. Gynaecology now has the fifth largest waiting list of all elective specialities across the UK, and it is the only speciality that solely affects women. Demand has grown dramatically, with 1.61 million gynaecology referrals in England between October 2024 and October 2025, up from 1.22 million between October 2019 and October 2020, an increase of around 24% (RCOG, 2026).

While waiting, women's conditions do not stand still. The Royal College of Obstetricians and Gynaecologists found that a quarter of women on waiting lists reported attending Accident and Emergency as a result of their symptoms, with more than one in ten of those women going on to have emergency interventions such as blood transfusions (RCOG, 2026). These are not women with mild, manageable discomfort. These are women in crisis, whose conditions have deteriorated while they waited for care that did not come.

Leanne Pickering's case is a perfect example of what frustration may lead to. She was told she suffered from endometriosis after having undergone twelve years of suffering, but still she had to face a two-year wait before getting treated by the NHS (BBC News, 2025). "They won't allow me to meet my endometriosis specialist unless I go through this checklist," said Leanne. "That can be really frustrating, especially when you've been diagnosed with endometriosis for many years."

Waiting, however, is not an inactive process. Women do not simply stay at home and remain untouched by their situations until their time comes. Instead, they go on living through pain, excessive bleeding, fatigue, and anxiety. They carry on with their lives, working, taking care of families, dealing with the demands of everyday life, while being forced to pay heed to their bodies. As mentioned by Tanya Simon-Hall, the founder of the Adeno Gang, which is an advocacy group for women suffering from adenomyosis, "Waiting lists are no abstract number these are lives on hold. For individuals with medical disorders such as adenomyosis and endometriosis, each passing month is associated with a deterioration of symptoms, relationships becoming tense, and opportunities being lost" (Simon-Hall, cited in RCOG, 2026).

And the postcode lottery ensures that this is made all the more difficult. The availability of diagnosis, treatments, and even pain relief is determined by one's postcode. There are certain locations where there are specialist centres for endometriosis as well as a well-established pathway of treatment, while other places only have standard gynaecological units with limited expertise. Patients find themselves having to move from pillar to post without a guide.

Fragmentation problem:

The biggest weakness of the existing system is fragmentation. Instead of flowing through an integrated system, women are shuffled around among separate services that are working independently and that individually have pieces of the story.

It usually takes more than one person to take care of the patient. The GP sends a referral to the gynaecologist. The ultrasound department takes pictures of the patient's body. If the first gynaecologist is not an expert in the matter, another gynaecologist can be called. Pain specialists can be contacted if the symptoms are very strong. A fertility specialist can be contacted if the problem affects conception. Colorectal surgeons are necessary if there are problems with the bowel. Urologists will be required if the bladder is involved in the condition.

For this woman in the middle of this fragmented system, the process consists of continuous repetitions. She shares her story with the GP, with the gynaecologist, with the ultrasound technician, with the pain specialist, and with the fertility consultant. Every single time, she is obliged to start from scratch, to tell about her symptoms, her medical history, and what other physicians have been doing for her. Every single time, she believes that this person will finally get it and see everything clearly.

India Weir, whose story was featured in the Royal College of Obstetricians and Gynaecologists' 2024 report 'Waiting for a Way

Forward,' shares this gruelling experience. Over a year after her surgery, India Weir was still waiting for the correct gynaecological support. "I frequently feel like I need to be an expert in myself," she said, "because if I don't, I don't know the next time I can contact someone or even access my records. I'm too mentally exhausted to give any attention to the things that I used to enjoy, such as meeting friends, spending time with family, or planning a vacation" (Weir, cited in RCOG, 2024).

This is not an inconvenience. It is a clinical hazard. Information that should be exchanged fails to make its way through. Test results are repeated or overlooked. Inconsistencies in advice are generated. The continuity of thought breaks down, and with it the ability to provide seamless care.

"Through my experience working for Cysters, I have witnessed the following description from many women who have been helped through our network: 'There is no communication between different health services, and this makes me give the same story repeatedly or even follow inconsistent advice, which could be frustrating. This has caused years of symptoms without having any support. As long as these basic aspects aren't taken care of, it is difficult for women to feel properly supported throughout the journey of care. " (Heera-Shergill, cited in RCOG, 2026).

Self-Coordination Burden

When the system cannot coordinate patient treatment, it places this burden upon women. And in truth, there is little choice in the matter. It becomes a means of survival in a healthcare system that does not connect itself. Women become investigators who piece together facts surrounding their diseases, which the doctors do not share with them. Women become managers who ensure that appointments are made, that records are requested and that referrals are completed. Women become lobbyists who campaign for further research into their ailments and symptoms.

This is work, and for the most part it remains invisible, as it takes place at home in evenings following work, during breaks in jobs that are themselves stressful, and in stolen time from family responsibilities. It requires effort, which chronically ill women simply cannot afford. And it doesn't even ensure success. All too often, women fall into a procrastination/rejection pattern.

The emotional toll on the body required for the coordination of one's body can be very great. Women have to become experts on their bodies to be heard. They educate themselves on clinical language through reading scientific journals, joining forums on the Internet, and educating themselves in order to appear as an educated patient. They even prepare as though attending a test to avoid being disqualified.

And when, having gone through all this effort, they encounter a doctor who won't listen to their concerns, who dismisses their fears as unnecessary worries, who suggests that they might just be feeling anxious, the consequences can be devastating. This isn't merely an unsuccessful visit. This is proof that the hours spent researching, preparing, and advocating for themselves were futile.

A story of Leanne Pickering having to fill out a "checklist" of actions before being referred to a specialist is a testament to how nonsensical this responsibility can be. She had already been diagnosed for years. She knew what she needed. Yet the system required her to jump through hoops designed for patients who had not yet been investigated, as if her history counted for nothing.

The requirement to self-coordinate is not distributed evenly. Women with greater financial resources, educational background, and social capital are better able to navigate the system, to push for what they need, and to access private care when the NHS fails them. Women without such resources are left to manage as best they can, which often places them even further behind. This division of care reinforces the inequalities already embedded in the system, producing a two-layered model in which those who can afford to pay do, and those who cannot remain on the list for years.

What the Strategy now promises

The Renewed Women's Health Strategy is explicit about the scale of the fragmentation problem, and it is explicit that the 2022 Women's Health Strategy failed to address it adequately (DHSC, 2026, p. 9). It commits to a set of structural changes that, if delivered, would genuinely alter what women experience in the next five years.

The most important of these is Action 28: a single point of access for all non-urgent gynaecology referrals, directing women to the right care community diagnostic centres, neighbourhood women's health services, or secondary care rather than requiring them to navigate a maze of separate services (DHSC, 2026, pp. 33–36). Action 29 commits to standardising care pathways for heavy periods, menopause and uro-gynaecology within three years, so that women are not required to attend multiple appointments in different places for tests and treatments. Action 30 funds a specialist centre in each NHS region for group-based approaches to women's health pathways, with early rollout focused on communities experiencing the highest levels of health need and inequity (DHSC, 2026, p. 36).

Action 36 is the one I find most interesting. It commits to prioritising menstrual problems including endometriosis, fibroids and adenomyosis as one of the first nine pathways established in NHS Online, the new virtual hospital launching in 2027 (DHSC, 2026, p. 38). In principle, this means that a woman in a rural area of Wales, or a woman who cannot take a day off work for an in-person appointment, will be able to access specialist care through a digital route. The value of this depends entirely on whether the virtual pathway connects her to an actual endometriosis specialist rather than to a generalist gynaecologist who does not know the condition well, a risk Leanne Pickering herself flagged in published commentary: "the biggest delays happen because patients aren't referred to the right people early enough" (Pickering, cited in BBC News, 2025).

The community shift is not a new idea. The Welsh Women's Health Hubs, announced in 2025 and scheduled for full rollout by March 2026, are an early pilot of the same principle (Welsh Government, 2026). Wales, Scotland and England are each experimenting with their own version. The Sunderland Women's Health Hub, a proof-of-concept site in the North East of England, has been evaluated by NIHR Applied Research Collaboration North East and North Cumbria. The evaluation found that for every £1 invested in the hub, £8 in benefits is generated over ten years (DHSC, 2026, p. 38, citing NIHR ARC NENC).

That is a real finding. It is also a reminder of something the NHS has known for a long time and has struggled to act on: community-based women's health care works. The question is whether the Renewed Strategy's commitments will be funded, staffed and sustained long enough for the model to reach every neighbourhood in the country, or whether, as has happened before, the ambition will dissolve into three years of consultation and then quietly recede.

I want to be clear about my view. I believe the Strategy is, on paper, the most serious attempt at reform I have seen in my career. I also believe that paper is the cheapest substance in Whitehall. The next chapter is about what happens inside the room where the real test of a strategy is conducted: the conversation between a woman and a clinician, where the question of whether she is heard is settled in nine minutes.

What women deserve

I want to end this chapter with a set of what I believe women have the right to expect from British gynaecological care in 2026, and what the Renewed Strategy has now committed, in part, to deliver.

A woman is entitled to a process that listens to her from day one rather than day ten.

She is entitled to flow through care pathways at the speed dictated by her condition, rather than being slowed down by a queue.

She is entitled to a patient record that travels with her so that she does not have to recount her history to seven different people in succession.

She is entitled to a single professional who takes ownership of her treatment.

She is entitled to a referral to a specialist when she needs one, based on her presenting symptoms and not a checklist applicable to some other individual.

She is entitled to services that do not vary depending upon how much money she has, where she lives, or what colour her skin happens to be.

None of these principles represents a radical agenda. These are fundamental conditions of an efficient public sector service. The fact that they read, in 2026, as ambitious is itself a measure of how far the system has fallen short.

The rest of this book is about how we reach that standard. It is also about what women can do, inside their own consultation rooms, while we wait.

※ ※ ※

CHAPTER FOUR

Communication, Trust, and Being Heard

Natalie's GP told her she could not have endometriosis.

The reason he gave, as she has since told Refinery29, was that she could not have endometriosis and must have fibroids instead, because — in his words — "it's what Black women get" (Refinery29, 2025). The doctor had pre-diagnosed her on sight. Natalie is Black British. She had been trying, at that point, for almost thirteen years to have her pain investigated. She told him, evenly, that her white mother had endometriosis, which the doctor took as neither medically relevant nor personally decisive. He still did not believe her (Refinery29, 2025).

Natalie was eventually diagnosed, at thirty-three, with endometriosis. She has had five surgeries since. She was, at a late stage of the process, told she was no longer eligible for NHS fertility treatment. The thirteen years she spent not being believed cost her the time within which options would have existed.

I want to begin this chapter with Natalie because her consultation room is the clearest place to stand to understand what I am going to talk about next. The failure she experienced was not a failure of information. Her GP had information. He had clinical training, access to the same NICE guidelines as every other GP in the country, and the full array of referral pathways at his disposal. What he did not have, what he had, in fact, substituted with a racialised assumption, was the willingness to hear the woman in front of him as a reliable narrator of her own body.

That willingness, or its absence, is what this chapter is about.

The architecture of the clinical encounter

The typical GP consultation in the United Kingdom lasts 9.2 minutes on average (Irving et al., 2017). Within this window, a doctor must establish rapport, take a history, consider differential diagnoses, conduct any necessary examination, agree on a management plan, and document the encounter. It is a demanding cognitive and interpersonal task, made more difficult by the pressure of a waiting room full of other patients with their own urgent needs.

For the woman presenting with gynaecological symptoms, these nine minutes are asked to do an impossible amount of work. She needs to explain to someone she has only just met the intricacies of her period, her pain, her bleeding, her toileting habits, her sexuality, and any worries she might have about her fertility. And she needs to do this, feeling all the awkwardness and discomfort that accompanies it. She needs to do it knowing that everything rests on this one short discussion.

According to the survey on reproductive health conducted in England in 2025, 61.9% of those questioned have had problems related to their periods (Palmer et al., 2025). There are only ten minutes on average per consultation to address these problems. This is not how one makes a careful assessment. This is rather making decisions using rules of thumb and quick judgment calls.

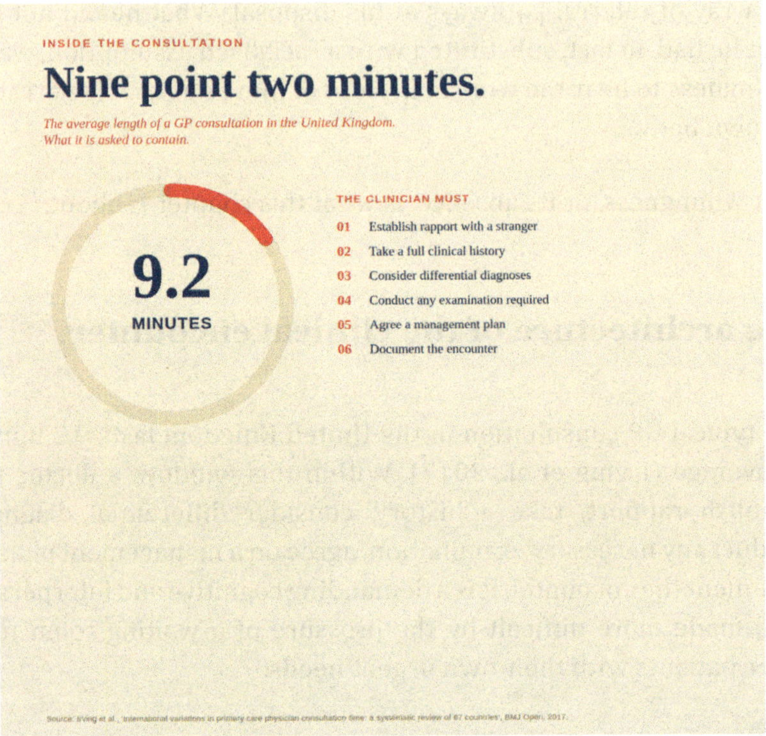

Figure 9. Nine point two minutes.

The medical gaze, which refers to the objective, clinical viewpoint from which the doctor examines his or her patient, is one that Beth Malory, an expert in health communication at University College London, highlights in her work (Malory, 2023). The medical gaze prevails when the condition lacks clear signs, requiring a great deal of research to make a diagnosis empirically. Anything a patient reports about his or her experience is considered subjective. Doctors prefer evidence they can visualise or measure, not what goes on inside a person's head.

Numerous cases that affect women's reproductive organs, such as endometriosis and fibroids, also fit within this description perfectly. Diagnosis of endometriosis requires a laparoscopy. A fibroid diagnosis is possible, but someone has to arrange for the scan first. Without the tests, only the patient's account stands as proof of what she experiences. Yet, unfortunately, in an extremely hurried setting like the nine-minute consultation, it is often seen as not enough.

Words of Dismissal

The words used to dismiss women's pain tend to be subtle, woven into the language used in clinical settings. In addition, many times, people do not even intend their statements as acts of dismissal but rather words of kindness and support. When a physician states, "Well, that's likely just something that is part of your life," the intention may actually be to reassure the patient. When a clinician tells his female patient to try to reduce stress, she may actually feel that he is doing her a favour. However, such words mean to the women whose pain is physical and very much real something entirely different.

According to the 2024 Nurofen survey on the Gender Pain Gap, 81% of women between the ages of 18 and 24 had their pains either downplayed or completely disregarded by healthcare professionals. In total, 62% of women felt that their pains were being downplayed in 2024 compared to the previous year, when only 35% did so. This increase is partly attributed to the fact that a quarter of all women began doubting themselves after feeling gaslighted medically.

The ramifications, however, do not end there. One-third of women in the survey said that their suffering being disregarded led to mental problems, increasing from a fourth in 2023. For a fifth, it affected their career choices. These are no trivial complaints. This is serious damage done, not by illness but by the treatment intended to cure it.

According to the Endometriosis UK survey, 78% of women who went on to get diagnosed have experienced doctors telling them "you're making a fuss about nothing". This percentage has gone up from 69% recorded in the previous survey conducted in 2020. This seems to indicate that although more is now known about endometriosis, patients continue to experience dismissive attitudes from doctors, which seem to be getting worse (Endometriosis UK, 2024). Just one woman in ten stated that her GP mentioned the possibility of endometriosis when discussing her symptoms in either her first or second visit.

Dismissal need not take the form of direct language. It may also involve silence on the part of the individual, such as failing to inquire into the effect of pain on one's everyday routine, failing to inquire into the nature and timing of any bleeding experienced, and immediately assuring the patient without checking for any other signs that could be cause for concern. Such behaviour sends a powerful non-verbal message, implying that whatever problems the patient is facing are simply not worth discussing.

The cumulative impact of discrimination

If the structure of the consultations and the language used to dismiss women make obstacles for all women, then these obstacles are greater, stronger, and more dangerous for Black women and other marginalised women. The communication breakdown is further aggravated by implicit biases, the subconscious preconceptions and prejudices that influence the way clinicians think about their patients.

In the 2024 submission to the Women and Equalities Select Committee, the NHS Race and Health Observatory was very clear about its views regarding reproductive healthcare: "Medical misogyny is further compounded by racism, leaving ethnic minority women at a disadvantage when it comes to reproductive health care" (NHS Race and Health Observatory, 2024). In particular, the submission referred to "several concerning trends, including stereotyping, not being heard, being disbelieved, a lack of education and awareness of barriers that racialised women face."

The numbers confirm it. For example, the Reproductive Health Survey for England 2025 revealed a significantly higher likelihood of developing reproductive morbidity among survey respondents from minority ethnic groups, especially those of the Black, Black British, Caribbean or African race/ethnicity (Palmer et al., 2025). Women of colour are more likely to have fibroids detected at a younger age, with larger and increased numbers of growths, and twice or three times more often suffer from related severe symptoms, such as pelvic pain and infertility. It is estimated that 80% of black women will have fibroids detected by age fifty, whereas 70% of white women will develop this condition.

However, although the condition is more prevalent and more severe among Black women, they experience more obstacles accessing treatment. Their symptoms are more often ignored, their diagnosis is delayed, and their prognosis is worse than that of other patients. This is not due solely to biological factors. Rather, it is the result of a health care system that perceives Black women's suffering as distinct from others', viewing their symptoms through a different, biased lens.

One of my fellow GPs, Dr Itunu Johnson-Sogbetun, has addressed the matter in her own personal experiences from within this phenomenon in her recent publication. Dr Johnson-Sogbetun mentions patients being told that their haemorrhage is "just what one would expect from African women," which is a great illustration of the role that cultural attitudes can play in healthcare provision (Johnson-Sogbetun, 2024). Patients are essentially being told that their body is different; their pain and their problems are expected; therefore, it does not warrant any further investigations.

The study by Perro et al. published in the British Medical Journal explicitly stated: "Racial discrimination and unconscious bias in the healthcare sector exacerbate obstacles to Black women accessing the menstrual health services they require" (Perro et al., 2024). The researchers argued that a holistic approach should be taken towards educating women about menstrual health, including the compulsory training of healthcare providers concerning the history of menstrual health knowledge and its effects on marginalised racial groups, along with more research on the incidence of menstrual disorders among Black women.

This is the field within which I have been working throughout my professional career. One of my own peer-reviewed research papers on the topic of barriers experienced by midwives while providing care to ethnic minority pregnant women with complications was published in Women and Birth (Chitongo et al., 2022). This paper confirmed all that I have outlined above: lack of communication, disruption of continuity of care, structural racism, and consequent erosion of trust once the woman felt she was not being listened to. In 2018, my work contributed to receiving the prestigious Mary Seacole Award, although I am bringing this up to provide additional background rather than to give extra credit for the arguments I put forward here.

Misunderstandings and interpretation issues

After implicit biases, there are the more prosaic but equally insidious issues of misunderstandings and interpretations. If both the physician and patient come from different cultural groups, then the possibilities for misunderstandings become manifold. What could be regarded by one as being within the range of "normal" might appear to the other to fall outside that range entirely.

One such paper published in the British Journal of General Practice is an example of how this process plays out. As some of the clinicians interviewed mentioned, the increased awareness of the menopause that is leading to these patients' visits may "not have been shared equally within communities" (Huang et al., 2023). "I cannot recall speaking to any woman of Black or Asian descent in relation to HRT; that's interesting," one healthcare professional stated. It is uncertain whether women from such ethnicities do not experience menopausal symptoms or whether they simply do not come forward with them.

There could be more than one reason for this behaviour, but there are certainly some other factors complicating the situation. The Healthwatch Berkshire report on women's health, based on conversations with 580 women, captured a direct example: "I'm very nervous to talk on the phone when I phone my doctor, I can't make them understand me easily, it's much better if I can speak to someone face to face" (Healthwatch Berkshire, 2023). For women who do not speak English as a first language, or who come from cultures where direct communication about intimate health matters is difficult, the telephone consultation increasingly common since the pandemic, adds another layer of challenge to an already difficult encounter.

The Renewed Women's Health Strategy acknowledges this problem directly. It commits to developing partnerships with voluntary organisations representing women most excluded from traditional services (Action 1: the Women's Voices Partnership), and to publishing an equity good practice guide to enable ICBs to reduce inequalities in heavy periods and menopause care (Action 34). Action 68 has already launched, through the National Institute for Health and Care Research, a new funding call focused on how best to improve communication around women's health across the life course, particularly in underserved or marginalised communities (DHSC, 2026, p. 57). These are welcome commitments. They also arrive after decades of research establishing exactly what needs to change. The question, again, is implementation.

What being heard looks like

If the picture painted so far is one of failure, it is worth asking: what does being heard actually look like? What does it feel like for a woman to walk out of a consultation and know that her pain has been taken seriously, her concerns respected, her testimony valued?

What it seems to be is a consultation lasting more than nine minutes, or a consultation where the clinician makes use of those nine minutes effectively.

What it seems to be is a clinician who poses open questions and heeds the answers without interruption or undue haste in reaching conclusions.

What it seems to be is a physician who brings up endometriosis and/or fibroids, who tells you what will happen next and gives you a referral, but at no point makes you feel that you have asked for too much.

What it seems to be is a clinician who accepts the limitations of the objectivity of scientific proof, saying, "I believe you, though there is nothing visible here in the scan." It seems to be someone who understands that pain does not need to be physically verified.

It looks like a partner rather than an authority figure delivering verdicts from on high.

The Patients Association's "Prescription for Outpatients" offers a vision of what this looks like at scale: supporting patient preparedness, embedding "what matters to you?" conversations, improving communication materials, integrating shared digital care plans, and reforming commissioning models to incentivise patient-centred approaches (Patients Association, 2024). These are achievable goals, supported by evidence, and informed by the experience of patients themselves.

The Renewed Strategy's Action 3 commits to developing Patient Reported Experience Measures (PREMs) for key women's health pathways, starting with gynaecological outpatient procedures within five years (DHSC, 2026, p. 20). Action 4 pilots "patient power payments", where the reimbursement NHS trusts receive is varied according to patient feedback on their experience of pain management. This is a genuinely novel policy. If it works, it creates the first financial incentive in the modern NHS for trusts to actually listen.

Action 7 commits to co-developing with women a standard of care for gynaecological procedures such as hysteroscopy, with particular attention to informed consent and choice of pain relief. The standard matters because one in three women currently reports severe pain scores of 7 or more out of 10 during NHS outpatient hysteroscopy without sedation (RCOG, 2024, cited in DHSC, 2026). This is a pain level that would not be accepted as routine in any other area of surgical care.

The right to be believed

And the problem of communication within women's healthcare is really one of trust, ultimately. Women cannot be trusted to know what is happening in their bodies, with their pain, with their experience. They are devalued, unheard, and invalidated. The problem does not fall equally on everyone, but rather falls harder on those already marginalised and disenfranchised. But it will impact all women, in some form or another, simply because that is how our system of healthcare works.

Belief is an essential component. Belief is what makes all else possible: investigations, diagnoses, treatment, and assistance. Lack of belief transforms the process into a game, a battle of credibility, leaving one feeling tired and hopeless. With belief, on the other hand, the interaction will be productive, an act of discovery together.

For the restoration of this right, transformation is needed on all fronts. Training needs to occur with respect to implicit bias and communication skills. Structures are needed for consultations that allow adequate listening time. Structures are needed for referrals that keep women's accounts alive throughout primary and secondary consultations. There is also a need for a culture that regards patient testimonies as knowledge in their own right, not as an inadequate stand-in for objectivity. Most importantly, there is a need for an acceptance of the expertise of those very women whose lives we are trying to improve.

The 81% of young women whose suffering was dismissed need more than that. The 78% of women with endometriosis who were called difficult need more than that. The Black women who have double or triple the chance of having fibroids but still find it more difficult to access healthcare need more than that. The women who leave appointments feeling invisible, ignored, and doubted need more than that.

They require a system that hears them out. They require clinicians who take them at their word. They require the right, which is so simple and yet so profound, to be heard.

The next chapter in this book is concerned with what the women have been up to all this time, in the interim period before their rights are fulfilled. The answer, as you may know if you belong to their ranks, is everything.

PART III

The Hidden Work Women Do

CHAPTER FIVE

Becoming Your Own Expert

There is a woman I know, in her early forties, who can tell you the surgical difference between a first-stage and fourth-stage endometriosis laparoscopy. She can tell you which of the eight drugs commonly prescribed for period pain work synergistically with which others. She can tell you which NHS trusts in the South East of England have accredited endometriosis specialist centres and which ones have closed their doors to new referrals. She can list, in order, the seven questions she has learned to ask in an appointment to avoid being sent home. She is not a clinician.

She is a librarian. She learned all of this because, for fifteen years, no doctor she saw would listen to her about the pain she was in.

I am going to call her Melissa, because that is not her name.

Melissa is one of thousands of British women who have done what the system required them to do to be treated: they have become expert patients. They have taught themselves what the clinicians would not. They have read the NICE guidelines because their GPs had not. They have made spreadsheets of their own symptoms, calibrated their own pain scales, researched which consultants in which hospitals are known to take women seriously, and arrived at appointments with the kind of preparation usually associated with job interviews.

I want to be careful how I write this chapter, because two true things sit uncomfortably next to each other. The first is that becoming your own expert is a profound injustice. It is not a thing a woman should have to do to be treated as a patient. It is a form of unpaid labour that the system extracts from women precisely because it has stopped performing its own clinical function, and the women best able to do it, educated, resourced, English-speaking, with time, are exactly the women who least need it. The ones who need it most are the ones least likely to be doing it.

The second true thing is that, at the time of writing, the system has not changed. Melissa is still what the system requires. Until the reforms promised by the Renewed Women's Health Strategy reach every consultation room in the country, some version of becoming your own expert will continue to be the practical route to being treated well. And it is worth being honest about what that takes.

This chapter is an attempt at both: to name the injustice, and to give you the tools if you need them.

What self-advocacy actually is

I want to clear away, first, a term that has come loose from its moorings.

Self-advocacy does not refer to any innate disposition. It is not "pushiness". Neither does it imply whether a woman has the proper kind of assertiveness, vocabulary, or upbringing. Self-advocacy is a set of procedures that can be learned.

Dr Karen Tang, the American gynaecologist authoring "It's Not

Hysteria," which has already touched the lives of many women, refers to self-advocacy as "the ability to partner with your healthcare provider to make sure all your questions are answered and all your worries are addressed" (Tang, 2024). This definition is important; the emphasis lies on partnership, not confrontation, which correctly defines self-advocacy as a professional skill in dealing with services, not as an ethics-based responsibility of sick women.

In essence, self-advocacy involves four different practices. Having worked with many women who have become competent in all four areas after having been within the system for a considerable time, I feel inclined to lay them out plainly, instead of trying to make them sound like some kind of mystical knowledge.

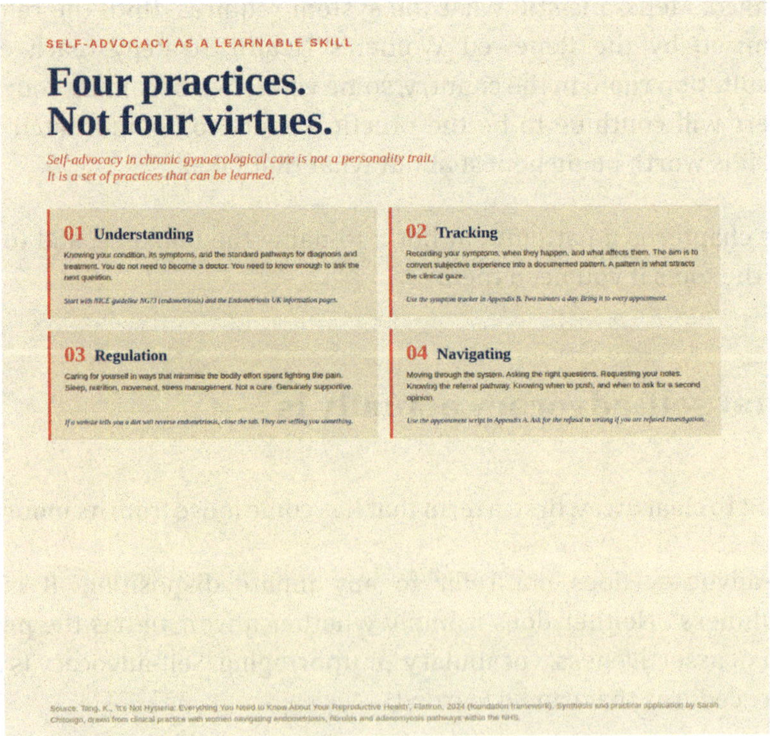

Figure 10. Four practices of self-advocacy.

The first practice is that of understanding. This entails gaining an understanding of your illness, its symptoms, and the standard procedures for diagnosing and treating it. This is not about becoming a doctor yourself. It is simply about being educated enough that you can clearly question the GP who suggests, "Let's try the Pill first and see if it makes a difference." The key points here are to understand whether the Pill in question is a combination pill or a mini-pill, and whether the treatment is supposed to target symptoms or the pathology itself.

The second strategy is tracking. Tracking entails recording your symptoms, when you experience them, and what effects they produce. I have provided more information about tracking in detail below, and you will find a worksheet in Appendix B. Tracking aims to turn a subjective observation into a documented pattern, since only a pattern attracts the clinical gaze. Emotionally, tracking provides something other than your own memory for the appointment, which will let you down, considering time constraints.

The third is self-care through regulation. Regulation involves taking care of yourself in a way that minimises bodily efforts spent fighting against the pain. It involves good sleep hygiene, proper nutrition, exercise, and stress management where possible. However, this does not constitute a cure for endometriosis or fibroids. And that, I want to emphasise, is a point that needs to be made quite clearly. If some social media account claims that you can reverse your condition by eating anti-inflammatory foods, they are just trying to sell you something. But there is good evidence that women who feel supported in their whole-body health cope better with chronic pelvic disease, and that some lifestyle adjustments make a genuine difference to inflammation, fatigue, and pain levels (Tang, 2024).

The fourth is navigating. This is the skill of moving through the system, the GP appointment, the referral, the specialist clinic, the imaging department, and the pharmacist. It involves asking the right questions, requesting copies of your notes, understanding the referral pathway, knowing when to push, and knowing when to seek a second opinion. It is, in effect, the work of being your own case manager.

None of these should be your job. Together, they are what currently passes as "being an engaged patient" in the British health service. Let us at least call the work what it is, and give women the tools to do it, while the system catches up.

Tracking, because it works

I want to say more about tracking because it is the single most effective thing a woman can do between now and her next appointment to change the outcome of that appointment.

A symptom tracker is not a diary. It is a structured record. The tracker I recommend, which appears in full in Appendix B, has columns for date, pain score out of ten, bleeding intensity, bowel and bladder symptoms, fatigue, mood, and impact on work, sex, and sleep. It takes perhaps ninety seconds a day to complete. It takes a month to develop data that can be reviewed within thirty seconds and conclusions drawn from it.

The value is simple enough. A woman reporting that "I have really bad periods" during a consultation is an impression that may be dodged easily. But a woman presenting a print-out that shows her pain scale readings of 7 or more for six days of each cycle, missing out on work for four days within three months, and experiencing pain with sexual intercourse on eleven occasions, has presented data. This transforms her into an evidence-bearing patient from just being one who has complaints. It is still the same narrative, but with new syntax that is readable through the clinician's gaze.

As one of the individuals who used to work with Aisha, a thirty-seven-year-old woman, I can vouch for her experience firsthand. As Aisha explains, "It took me years to convince doctors that my period pains were different from the usual pains. However, it was difficult because I lacked any data that would help me prove my point. After I started using the tracker, however, things changed. I could point to certain dates where I felt unable to leave my bed and certain weeks when I skipped work because of my period pains."

This is what happens in the case of the tracker. It doesn't change anything about the pain itself; rather, it renders the pain legible.

One might wonder whether digital apps, such as Clue, Flo, and other similar apps, might be helpful in this regard. It seems highly likely that the NHS Online virtual hospital, due to be launched in 2027, will have some integrated tracking applications (DHSC, 2026). In the meantime, however, a single-page tracker accompanied by a pen is enough.

Pain and the body as a system

Let me say something about pain now and the nature of its behaviour when unmanaged. This chapter has nothing to do with self-blame. It is about gaining insight because understanding gives one a foothold.

Chronic pain is not just an undistorted message received in the brain by the damaged tissues sending it out. Pain is processed, enhanced and controlled by the nervous system. In the case where pain lasts for months or years without any remedy, as seen in endometriotic and fibroid pain, there is an increase in sensitivity in the nervous system itself. There develops what is known as central sensitisation, whereby the pain threshold is lowered, pain levels are increased and stimuli that would otherwise not be painful become so (Moseley and Butler, 2015). However, this is not made-up pain but rather a physiological one, which is real and measurable. What this implies is that chronic pelvic pain, once it has been initiated, will exist beyond the physical lesions. The surgical removal of endometriosis does not guarantee an automatic relief of pain.

This is important in practical terms for two reasons.

First, it represents the medical basis for how some women with less visible disease suffer severe pain symptoms, whereas some women who have extensive disease experience fewer symptoms. There is no clear correlation between the severity of disease and pain symptoms (Chapron et al., 2019). Historically, this was viewed as a basis for disbelief among women who experienced "excessive" pain symptoms compared to the results of their imaging tests. The reverse inference is the accurate one. Pain experienced by a woman does not necessarily have to correlate with imaging findings to be legitimate.

Second, it means that pain management, as opposed to disease management, is a legitimate clinical priority in its own right. Pelvic physiotherapy, pain neuroscience education, graded movement, and, where appropriate, pain-modulating medications can reduce the central sensitisation component of chronic pelvic pain even when the underlying disease remains (Moseley and Butler, 2015). The Renewed Women's Health Strategy's Action 8 commits to working with the Getting It Right First-Time programme on secondary care gynaecology and chronic pain, specifically to improve standards in chronic pelvic pain management (DHSC, 2026). This is long overdue.

The practical implication for a woman reading this is: if your pain has persisted for years, ask about pelvic physiotherapy. Ask about pain management services. The answer in many NHS areas will be "we don't have a service for that". Note the answer. It is part of the evidence base for why you may need to push harder, and it is part of the evidence base for what needs to change nationally.

Food, inflammation, and the evidence

I want to be cautious here because this territory is thick with misinformation. The wellness industry has monetised endometriosis and fibroids to a degree that I find embarrassing on behalf of medicine, which has left the field open for it by refusing to engage with lifestyle as legitimate support. Neither the cult of the "endo diet" nor the medical establishment's instinct to dismiss all nutritional thinking is correct. The honest picture is in between.

The evidence for anti-inflammatory dietary patterns, not specific diets, but broad patterns reducing inflammatory markers in women with endometriosis, is reasonable, though not conclusive. A Mediterranean-style pattern, with regular consumption of oily fish, leafy vegetables, whole grains, olive oil, and reduced consumption of ultra-processed foods and red meat, is the pattern that appears most consistently in the literature (Ott et al., 2012; Parazzini et al., 2013). Specific foods with plausible anti-inflammatory effects for pelvic pain include fatty fish (salmon, sardines, mackerel), walnuts and flaxseeds, leafy greens, turmeric, ginger, and berries. Foods that consistently appear to worsen symptoms in many women include alcohol, ultra-processed foods, and high-sugar foods.

None of this is a cure. None of this replaces clinical treatment. For some women, dietary changes make no perceptible difference; for others, they reduce pain intensity and fatigue meaningfully. If you have the resources to try, it is worth trying.

What I want you not to do is take on another form of self-blame. If you are reading a forum that suggests your endometriosis would disappear if only you ate the right things, please close the tab. Endometriosis is a systemic disease with a complex aetiology that includes immune, endocrine, genetic and environmental factors (Chapron et al., 2019). The notion that it is caused by dietary sin is not supported by evidence and is actively harmful to women already carrying years of self-recrimination about their bodies.

The Renewed Strategy does not name dietary interventions specifically, but its Action 64 commits to a new programme to improve education for girls about their menstrual health, investing £1 million from this year in schools and community settings (DHSC, 2026). This is welcome. It is also an acknowledgement that, as a country, we have failed to provide girls with the basic biological literacy to understand their own bodies. We should not be surprised when, a decade later, those girls turn into women who are easy prey for wellness misinformation.

The shadow of access

I want to step back for a moment, because everything I have said in this chapter comes with a caveat that matters more than anything else in it.

Self-advocacy, in all four of its forms, is easier for some women than others. It is easier if you are a native English speaker. It is easier if you have time, which in practice means either financial resources or supportive employment. It is easier if you have the cultural confidence to challenge a doctor, which is itself distributed unequally along lines of race, class, and age. It is easier if you have a GP who is at least neutral rather than actively hostile. It is easier if you live in a part of the country with a specialist centre within travelling distance.

This is why, for all that I believe the tools in this chapter and the appendices are useful and I do I refuse to offer them as a solution to the systemic problem. If the NHS requires women to become their own experts to be treated, then the NHS is failing. A two-tier system in which articulate, resourced women receive decent care, and everyone else waits, is not a public health service in any sense that the 1948 founders of the NHS would recognise.

I say this with particular care for the women most likely to be failed. If you are a woman for whom English is a second language, or who has been treated with suspicion by doctors because of her accent or ethnicity, or who has not had the education to comfortably challenge a clinician, please know that your inability to become your own expert is not a failure on your part. It is a reflection of a system that should never have required it.

The rest of this book, and in particular Chapter Ten, is about the community structures that exist to support women who cannot do this work alone. You do not have to do this alone. And in a better country, you would not have to do it at all.

The appointment, revisited

I want to end this chapter with a practical scene. You have a GP appointment next Tuesday. You are going to describe, for what feels like the tenth time, a pain that the last nine clinicians have chosen to reassure rather than investigate. What, if anything, is different this time?

Three things, if you have used this chapter.

First, you have a tracker. You have a printed page showing the last two or three cycles in the data. Pain scores. Days missed. Bleeding intensity. You hand it across the desk in the first minute of the appointment. The act of handing it over changes the register of the conversation.

Second, you have a script. The full version is in Appendix A. The two lines I want you to have in your head are these:

"If it isn't endometriosis or fibroids, what else could this be, and what investigation would rule it out?"

"Could you document in my notes today that I asked for an investigation and was advised against it?"

The first question moves the clinician from reassurance mode into differential-diagnosis mode, which is where they are trained to be at their most rigorous. The second question converts the encounter into a documented one, and documentation changes what happens next in ways I have seen repeatedly in my practice. Most GPs, faced with the prospect of a written record of their refusal, will reconsider.

Third, you have information. You know, from reading this book, what the reassurance trap looks like. You know that the 2022 Endometriosis UK survey found 78% of women diagnosed with endometriosis were told they were making a fuss about nothing. You know that the Secretary of State for Health and Social Care has put the phrase "medical misogyny" in a government document (DHSC, 2026). You know, in other words, that what has happened to you is a pattern, and you can name it.

If the appointment still goes badly, and it may, you are not without options. You can request a second opinion. You can request a female GP or a GP with an interest in women's health. You can contact the practice manager in writing. You can, in England, complain via the practice's Patient Advice and Liaison Service, and if that fails, escalate to the Parliamentary and Health Service Ombudsman. All of this is hard. All of it is also your right.

The NICE guideline on endometriosis, updated in 2024, is clear: women with persistent symptoms of endometriosis should be referred to a gynaecologist (NICE, 2024). The Royal College of General Practitioners' learning module on endometriosis, updated in 2025, is clear about the same thing. If your GP refuses, they are not following the national guideline. That is a statement of fact, not a statement of emotion. You are allowed to say it.

Melissa, again

I began this chapter with Melissa, the librarian who learned more about endometriosis than some of the doctors who saw her. I would like to finish by saying something that she said to me, which I will always remember.

The day she got her laparoscopy, when she was almost forty years old, the doctor who gave her the diagnosis looked at her with slight professional amazement and asked her how she knew so much about her disease. And she told him. "Twenty years," she said. "Twenty years and about fifteen GPs." There was a pause, and then he said, "I'm sorry it took so long."

She said she cried in her car after that. Not from relief. From anger. She had wanted to hear those words for twenty years, and nobody had said them, and she had had to build an entire education to get to the room where someone finally would.

She also told me something else. She said that the worst of it was not the pain. The worst of it was the feeling that she had been wrong about her own body for two decades, and having to unlearn that. Having to learn, in her forties, that her witness had been reliable all along.

If you take nothing else from this chapter, take that. You are the reliable witness. You have always been the reliable witness. The system is what needs to change, and until it does, the work you do to be heard is not evidence that you are difficult. It is evidence that you are paying attention.

It is also, and I do not say this lightly, part of how the system changes.

Each woman who demands, who carries the tracker, who poses the question, who rejects the reassurance, contributes to the pressure, making the system adapt. The consultant of Melissa heard her story. He could very well think about it again when he sees another woman sitting across from him. What you are doing here is not just for yourself.

The following chapter is on the price of that work. It is the one which took me the most difficulty to write.

※ ※ ※

CHAPTER SIX

The Emotional Cost of Self-Advocacy

Lupita Nyong'o appeared on the TODAY show in February 2026 and said something which I have found myself constantly considering since then.

It wasn't something about waiting lists, surgery, or the inadequacies of the existing treatment protocols, although she is a passionate campaigner for all those things. No, it was about her personal emotional reaction to the news. "I felt shame," she confided in the interviewer's ear. "What did I do wrong to bring them upon me? And I felt very alone and quite terrified about what they might mean for my ability to have children in the future" (TODAY, 2026).

She is an Oscar winner. She can consult any doctor she wants, anywhere around the world. She is famous. She is articulate. She has a wonderful career, a supportive family and religious faith to rely upon. She has had seventy-seven fibroids throughout her life, most of which are currently more than fifty. And the first thing she described, in the interview that launched her public advocacy, was shame.

If Lupita Nyong'o felt shame, I want you to understand how that refracts. If a woman with every advantage the world can offer, still, at the point of diagnosis, asks herself what she did to cause it, then the shame around these diseases is not a personal failing of any one patient. It is a cultural condition. It is something we have done, collectively, over generations, to women's bodies and to women's understanding of their bodies.

This chapter is about what self-advocacy costs, and what it costs beyond the obvious. The obvious cost is time and money. The harder cost is psychological, and it is borne by almost every woman who has fought to be diagnosed, and it does not go away the day a clinician finally says the word.

The shame that is not yours

Let me begin where Lupita began. Shame.

I have sat with women who described feeling ashamed of their bodies for producing these diseases, ashamed of their pain for being so disproportionate to what doctors could see, ashamed of their emotional reactions to pain, ashamed of needing time off work, ashamed of not being able to have sex with their partners, ashamed of difficulty conceiving, ashamed of having a hysterectomy, ashamed of not having a hysterectomy, ashamed of asking for help, ashamed of asking for more help, ashamed of being the kind of patient doctors might describe as difficult.

It is an irrational shame, but it is not random either. It is the expected consequence of a society that teaches girls and women to see their pain in menstruation as a personal responsibility. As Tanya Simon-Hall, the founder of Adeno Gang, a support group for adenomyosis patients, aptly puts it, "Long waiting lists are not merely statistics; they are lives put on hold." And then came her understated yet poignant remark,

"When you have conditions such as adenomyosis and endometriosis, each passing month means more pain, worse symptoms, deteriorating relationships, and lost chances" (Simon-Hall, cited in RCOG, 2026).

Missed chances. The promotion you stepped back from because you could not be reliable enough to take it. The relationship that ended because you could not explain, even to the person who loved you, why some weeks you did not want to be touched. The pregnancy that did not happen, or did not hold. The Christmas you spent in bed instead of at the table. The friendships that quietly faded because you stopped saying yes to anything. These are not the kind of losses a doctor asks about, and they do not appear in any clinical record. They are, between them, the largest part of what these conditions actually cost.

Hayley, whose mango-sized fibroid was only detected through ultrasound in her early thirties, recalls that her initial response to the discovery was one of relief rather than fear (Endometriosis UK, 2024). This is precisely how the wound to the heart feels. A woman does not have to be diagnosed with a tumour to feel better about believing her experience with her body.

Performing Credibility

In Chapter Two, I touched on being an expert in yourself. What was not captured in the discussion was the price paid for such expertise.

Self-advocacy, for most endometriosis patients and fibroid sufferers, does not occur in a single instance. This is rather an ongoing process. Whenever you meet another doctor, go for an appointment, or seek a new health care service, you need to be prepared with the right language, tone, and symptom history. The minute you lose it, let one tear flow, ask one assertive question, and the whole discussion may fall within the realm of a doctor's mindset called "anxious patient," from which it is extremely hard to break free.

It is an exhaustion that is hard to describe to anyone who has not lived inside it. It is the exhaustion of impression management, in a setting where the consequence of getting your tone wrong is that your pain is not treated. It is a form of labour that endometriosis and fibroids patients perform on top of being ill.

Such an activity creates chronic stress and thus brings about biological implications. Chronic activation of the hypothalamic-pituitary-adrenal axis in the body is linked to immune disorders, inflammation, and heightened pain (McEwen, 2017). In essence, the labour involved in getting recognition exacerbates the illness. There is an irony to the fact that the labour of self-advocacy leads to symptoms that require advocacy in the first place.

The Nurofen Gender Pain Gap Survey in 2024 revealed one aspect of this cycle through its statistics. Almost a third of women surveyed said that being made to feel like their pain was not important led to them feeling mentally unwell. Around a fifth of women indicated that their careers had been impacted by their pain experiences. One in four said that they began doubting themselves and their own sanity because their pain was continually invalidated and discounted (Nurofen, 2024). And this number, I believe, is the most alarming of all.

Isolation

It is no fun to suffer alone at the best of times, but unproven and undiagnosed chronic pelvic pain is solitude with added walls.

This is the way women relate it to me, time after time. Your friends are sick of asking how you are doing because the response never changes, and you have no idea how to cope with it. Your loved ones love you and want to help, but the distance created by an ongoing illness proves difficult to bridge. At work, your colleagues think the problem is a lack of commitment and reliability. And your family tells you to pull yourself together and perhaps here we are seeing the older generation of women, who suffered in silence, come to life again.

The Internet and social media platforms have proven invaluable for many women suffering from chronic health conditions like endometriosis, fibroids, and adenomyosis. This has enabled them to connect with others in similar situations, share information, and validate their personal experiences. While one needs to be fair in such statements, since there is also potential for spreading misinformation online, the importance of connecting with other women, even if it is 2 in the morning, and realising that they are facing similar issues that have been brushed off by their doctors, cannot be underestimated. It is usually the first time when women feel they have been heard.

These are not marginal groups. These are, for many women I know personally, the main sources of information, emotional support, and practical guidance. The reason why such organisations exist is that the official health care system failed in its job. The structure that should have been created by the NHS decades ago was created by people outside the healthcare system. Chapter Ten goes into further detail on all of these organisations. For the moment, it is enough just to point out their presence as proof of how great the need is.

Second sentence by Lupita Nyong'o

I would like to go back to Lupita Nyong'o, who, during her TODAY show interview, gave us something unique: a detailed explanation of the emotional path of a woman through a fibroid diagnosis, in the eloquent words of someone who understood the experience.

After the shame, she described isolation. After the isolation, she described something else. "I've found community," she said. "I've locked arms with women who have been fighting this fight for a long time" (TODAY, 2026). She then committed herself publicly to the Foundation for Women's Health's fibroid research fund and to advocacy for the U-FIGHT Act in the United States, which is seeking $150 million in research funding over five years (Complex, 2026).

I have watched what has happened in the two months since that interview. British women who had not previously felt able to talk about their fibroids have started to. Black women in the UK have said, in social media posts and in messages sent to Cysters and similar organisations, that they saw themselves on television for the first time. Clinicians have told me, quietly, that they have had more first-time fibroid consultations this spring than they had in the previous year. One interview, conducted by one powerful woman, has made an impact.

This is what I mean by the struggle on the level of public consciousness. Policy change is important. Guidelines are important. Access to services is important. But so is the very basic statement of one woman being vocal enough to say, "I'm in pain; I know I'm not alone, and I will speak up about my experience."

Lupita's power is not needed for this to have relevance. One woman going to her GP and explaining how the reading of her symptoms has confirmed that she may be suffering from endometriosis and that she needs to be evaluated for the condition is changing things, one conversation at a time. One woman sharing her story and saying how she was correct all along with her sister, her friend, and her child is changing things. These countless acts are the ones that lead to the implementation of the Renewed Strategy.

It is, moreover, something that helps make the price emotionally worth paying. Shared grief is not the same as solitary grief; anger aimed at an impersonal system is not the same as anger pointed inward. The women whom I have known who are able to have the healthiest relationship with their diagnoses are, without exception, those who have managed to find a community and become part of something greater than themselves and their particular situation. This is equally true whether they are still awaiting treatment or are in the midst of experiencing the pain.

Mental health is a genuine clinical concern here.

It is time I made a point clear, one that clinicians generally refrain from making because they do not want their patients to feel like they are suggesting their gynaecological pain is all in their mind.

The burden of mental illness among women who suffer from endometriosis, fibroids, and adenomyosis is a real burden and needs to be addressed clinically in its own right. There is no indication that it is a condition of imagination, but rather a logical outcome of untreated physical pain.

Research on endometriosis and mental health shows elevated rates of depression, anxiety, and post-traumatic stress symptoms in women with the condition, particularly those who experience long diagnostic delays (Chen et al., 2016; van Barneveld et al., 2022). The 2023 Adult Psychiatric Morbidity Survey in England found that around one in four women has a common mental health condition, compared with around one in seven men (NHS England, 2024). Women are almost twice as likely as men to have an eating disorder, more likely to have attempted suicide or self-harmed, and more likely to have post-traumatic stress disorder (DHSC, 2026, citing NHS England). There is also increasing recognition of the links between female hormones and mental health, in conditions such as premenstrual dysphoric disorder (PMDD), which has itself historically been dismissed as "just hormonal" (Tang, 2024).

The Renewed Strategy's Action 49 commits to improving mental health support for women and girls, with NHS Talking Therapies expansion targeting 915,000 completed courses of treatment by March 2029, and with community mental health centres providing trauma-informed care (DHSC, 2026). Access to these services remains patchy, and the wait is often long. If you are struggling with your mental health alongside your physical symptoms, please do not take on the additional belief that your distress is a weakness. It is not. It is a rational response to an irrational situation, and it is treatable in its own right.

Please also know that if you are in crisis, the Samaritans line (116 123, free from any phone in the UK) is available twenty-four hours a day. If you are thinking about harming yourself, please tell someone. The phrase "medical misogyny" in a government document does not help a woman at midnight in a bathroom. A person, at a phone, does.

Partners, families, and the people who love us

I want to say a word to the people who love women with these conditions, because if there is one constituency I wish read this book alongside the women themselves, it is them.

Partners of women with endometriosis, fibroids and adenomyosis often feel helpless. They watch their partner in pain, they see the medical system fail her, they do not know what to say, and they do not know what to do. Some respond by becoming advocates alongside her; some respond by withdrawing, because the helplessness is unbearable; some respond by quietly suggesting, out of love rather than malice, that perhaps she is making a bit too much of it. All of these are human responses. Only one of them helps.

What helps, in my clinical experience, is belief. It is the single most important thing a partner can give. Belief that the pain is real, belief that the dismissal has been wrong, belief that the woman's instinct about her own body is worth listening to. A partner who walks into a GP appointment with her and says, on the record, "I have watched her be in this pain for six months, and I am concerned it is not being investigated", changes the dynamic of the room. Abby Norman, in her memoir Ask Me About My Uterus, described how she was only taken seriously when accompanied by her boyfriend, who confirmed that her sexual performance was, indeed, compromised (Norman, 2018). That story is ten years old and still true. The architecture of the consultation room has historically given a male voice a corroborative weight that a woman's own voice does not have. Use this unfairness, for now, if you have it available.

Parents of teenagers who are describing disabling period pain: please believe them. The 2025 Reproductive Health Survey for England found that more than a third of women aged 16 to 24 described their periods as severely painful (Palmer et al., 2025). This is not normal for a young woman. It is a sign that something may need investigation. If your GP reassures, push for a referral. Your daughter's future fertility, her educational outcomes, and her mental health may depend on it.

Friends, colleagues, siblings: the most useful thing you can do is not offer solutions. The most useful thing is to make clear that you believe her, that you see the effort she is making, and that you are available. A woman with chronic pelvic pain does not need you to fix it. She needs you not to require her to perform wellness for your comfort.

The long game

I want to end with something practical, because this is not a chapter that should end in elegy.

The emotional cost of self-advocacy is real. It is not a reason to stop. It is a reason to build in what sustains you alongside the work.

In my clinical experience, the women who last longest in the fight, the ones who reach their diagnosis, continue to advocate for better treatment, and become community supporters for other women, have three things in common. They have at least one person they trust to believe them unconditionally, a medical professional or otherwise. They have a practice of some kind that reconnects them with their body in a context other than pain, whether that is swimming, knitting, gardening, prayer, or just walking in the park. And they have a community of other women with similar experiences, whether online or in person, that gives them both practical information and the gift of being understood without explanation.

You do not need all three at once. One is a start. Over time, adding the others is protective.

And when you can, if you can, tell your story. Not because your story is owed to the public, because it is not. But because each story told moves the needle, and because the women coming up behind you, the fourteen-year-old missing school, the seventeen-year-old wondering whether this is her life now, will grow up in a world differently shaped by what you have said.

The next two chapters are about inequality, and about the specific ways the system has failed Black, Asian, and marginalised women. It is the strongest section of this book. It is also, by some distance, the section I have thought about longest, because it is the territory of my own professional life. I want to be clear: what follows is not an appendix to the argument. It is the centre of it.

PART IV

Inequality and Experience

CHAPTER SEVEN

When Care Isn't Equal

I want to start this chapter with two statements of fact, and then ask you to hold them next to each other.

The first is from the 2025 Reproductive Health Survey for England, the largest study ever conducted of women's reproductive health in this country. It found that Black women, Black British women, Caribbean women and African women had the highest odds of reporting reproductive morbidity of any ethnic group surveyed (Palmer et al., 2025).

The second is from Refinery29's 2025 feature on Black women and endometriosis in the UK. It documents Natalie's consultation with a GP who told her she could not have endometriosis because "it's what white women get." Natalie is Black British. Her white mother had endometriosis. She told him. He still did not believe her. She was finally diagnosed at thirty-three, after thirteen years (Refinery29, 2025).

These two statements are not in tension. They are the same statement. Black women in the UK have the highest rates of poor reproductive health. Black women in the UK also have the worst access to diagnosis and care. This is not an unfortunate coincidence. It is a system working exactly as it has been designed to work or not designed at all, which amounts to the same thing. A system that cannot distinguish between two conditions because it has decided, in advance, which condition a Black body is entitled to have is a system that is actively producing the inequality it then describes in data.

This is the chapter I have been preparing to write for most of my career. Some of the evidence I am going to cite in it is my own.

The fibroid paradox, and what it does

Fibroids are the most common benign tumours of the female reproductive tract. Approximately 80% of Black women will develop them by the age of fifty, compared to 70% of white women. Black women tend to develop fibroids earlier, in greater numbers, and with more severe symptoms (Stewart et al., 2017; Scottish Government, 2026; Katon et al., 2023).

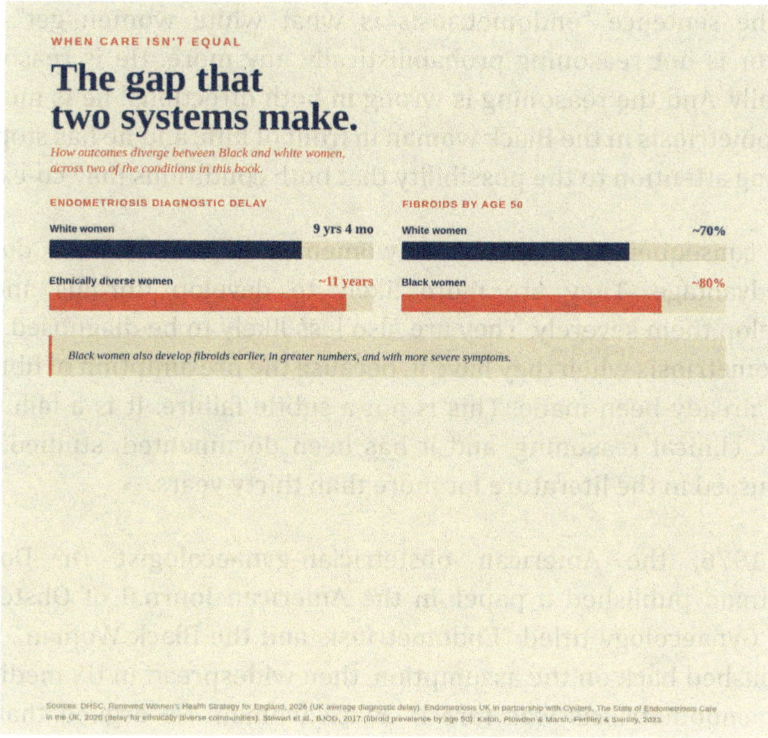

Figure 11. When care isn't equal: the gap that two systems make.

Endometriosis, by contrast, has historically been underdiagnosed in Black women. A 2019 systematic review in BJOG found Black women were roughly half as likely as white women to be diagnosed with endometriosis (odds ratio 0.49, 95% confidence interval 0.29–0.83), based on sixteen studies (Bougie et al., 2019). Asian women, by contrast, were 1.63 times more likely to receive an endometriosis diagnosis than white women (Bougie et al., 2019).

What this produces, in the consultation room, is what I call the fibroid paradox. A Black woman in pain is treated by many clinicians as statistically more likely to have fibroids than endometriosis. That statistical reasoning then hardens, in some clinicians, into a presumption. The presumption shows up, as it showed up for Natalie, as the sentence "endometriosis is what white women get". The doctor is not reasoning probabilistically any more. He is reasoning racially. And the reasoning is wrong in both directions: he is missing endometriosis in the Black woman in front of him, and he has stopped paying attention to the possibility that both conditions may co-exist.

The consequence is that Black women in the UK suffer a double disadvantage. They are more likely to develop fibroids and to develop them severely. They are also less likely to be diagnosed with endometriosis when they have it, because the presumption of fibroids has already been made. This is not a subtle failure. It is a failure of basic clinical reasoning, and it has been documented, studied, and discussed in the literature for more than thirty years.

In 1976, the American obstetrician-gynaecologist Dr Donald Chatman published a paper in the American Journal of Obstetrics and Gynaecology titled "Endometriosis and the Black Woman". In it, he pushed back on the assumption, then widespread in US medicine, that endometriosis was rare in Black women. He argued that the pelvic pain of Black women was being systematically misdiagnosed most commonly as pelvic inflammatory disease, an infection-related condition then strongly associated in medical culture with sexual activity, and therefore freighted with racialised judgement. He suggested that the early descriptions of endometriosis as a disease of the "well-dressed" and "trim" middle-class white woman had shaped who was considered eligible for the diagnosis (Chatman, 1976; Buttram, 1979).

That was half a century ago. Natalie was told she could not have endometriosis because she was Black in 2012. The presumption has survived the evidence by five decades.

Maternal mortality and the argument that connects them

I want to bring in something that is sometimes treated as a separate subject, because it is not.

Black women in the UK are nearly three times more likely to die in pregnancy or childbirth than white women. Asian women are almost twice as likely (MBRRACE-UK, 2024). Babies born to Black women are more than twice as likely to die in their first year compared to babies born to white women (DHSC, 2026, p. 8).

These statistics are staggering on their own. What matters for this chapter is that they arise from the same underlying mechanisms as the delay in endometriosis diagnosis and the dismissal of fibroid pain. They are produced by a system that does not hear Black women's descriptions of their own bodies. In maternal care, that failure shows up as symptoms of haemorrhage or pre-eclampsia being normalised until it is too late. In gynaecological care, it shows up as a decade's delay in diagnosis, or as a woman being sent home repeatedly with pain that turns out to be cancer.

I have spent much of my research career on this. My 2022 paper in Women and Birth, co-authored with colleagues at Middlesex University, examined midwives' insights into the common barriers in providing effective perinatal care to women from ethnic minority groups with high-risk pregnancies (Chitongo et al., 2022). We found communication gaps, cultural assumptions, structural racism, and the continuing reality that a Black woman in an NHS delivery suite was statistically less likely to have her concerns believed in the crucial minutes of an emergency. My Mary Seacole Award in 2018 was for a body of research on exactly this territory. I mention this because it matters for credibility and because I want you, reader, to know that what I am telling you about the situation of Black women in British healthcare is not a secondary interest for me. It is the through-line of my professional life.

What I learned, painfully, is that the patterns I was documenting in maternity care are the same patterns that produce the outcomes described in the paragraphs above. A GP who does not believe a Black woman's description of her period pain in 2024 will grow into, or be trained by, or work alongside, a midwife or obstetrician who does not believe a Black woman's description of her contractions in 2028. These are not separate problems. They are the same problem, staged in different rooms.

Parliament, finally

On the 5th of March 2026, the House of Commons held a debate on endometriosis and fibroids as part of the consideration of the Women's Health Strategy. It was the most sustained parliamentary attention these conditions have received in UK history.

Members of Parliament rose, one after another, to speak about their constituents. One MP described the opening of the debate in language that I want to quote directly, because it is unusual for the floor of the Commons: "Endometriosis, fibroids and related gynaecological conditions ruin the lives of millions of women, yet these conditions remain undiagnosed, misdiagnosed, dismissed or mistreated within the health system. Women are told to shut up and stop complaining. We are fobbed off. We experience shameful delays. We are left in pain" (Hansard, 2026).

Another MP directly named the racial disparity: "Black women are disproportionately affected, and often face barriers to timely and compassionate care. This is also the case for ethnically diverse women with endometriosis, as highlighted in the Endometriosis UK report" (Hansard, 2026). A third cited the twenty or so women MPs currently in the House who, by simple statistical distribution, would themselves be living with endometriosis.

This is nothing. A Parliament that names the disease, quantifies its prevalence, acknowledges the racial inequality, and then puts all of it on the public record is a Parliament that has been forced, by advocacy and by data, to take it seriously. The same debate contributed to the political weight behind the Renewed Women's Health Strategy published six weeks later. There is no way that the foreword that the Secretary of State wrote on "medical misogyny" came out of the blue. It came after a long-running campaign spearheaded by activists such as Emma Cox from Endometriosis UK, Neelam Heera-Shergill from Cysters, and Tanya Simon-Hall from the Adeno Gang, along with MPs who were listening to them.

I want to be honest again: a Hansard record is not a diagnosis in a woman's file. The women in this chapter are still waiting. But the shift from invisibility to named-in-Parliament is the first condition of everything else. Until the conditions were named, nothing could be built.

What the Strategy commits to, specifically on equity

The Renewed Women's Health Strategy has an explicit equity thread, and I want to describe it precisely, because it is the benchmark against which the government now has to deliver.

Action 1 establishes the Women's Voices Partnership in 2026–27, with an explicit focus on organisations representing women most excluded from traditional services. Cysters, Black Womxn's Health, Five X More, Jamii, and similar organisations are likely to be among the groups brought into national policy-making for the first time (DHSC, 2026, p. 19).

Action 20 commits to co-developing care and support between pregnancies for marginalised communities with the NIHR Maternity Disparities Consortium, with an initial goal of reversing the worsening decline in preconception folic acid supplement use by the end of 2027, and delivering the UK's first blueprint for such care by 2030 (DHSC,

2026, p. 28).

Action 30 funds regional specialist centres for group-based approaches to high-volume women's health pathways, heavy periods, contraception, uro-gynaecology, and menopause, with early rollout targeted at communities experiencing the highest levels of health need and inequity (DHSC, 2026, p. 36).

Action 34 commits to publishing an equity good practice guide to help Integrated Care Boards reduce inequalities in heavy periods and menopause care specifically, identifying these as conditions that disproportionately affect women from ethnic minority backgrounds and those in the 20% most deprived areas (DHSC, 2026, p. 37).

Most importantly, the Strategy commits to setting an explicit target to close the Black and Asian maternal mortality gap, informed by the Amos Investigation, whose findings are due in June 2026 (DHSC, 2026, p. 14, p. 47). This is the first time in my professional life that a government has committed to a specific equity target on maternal mortality.

I will believe it when I see the target delivered. I have been wrong before, in optimistic directions, about government commitments in this territory. But on paper, this is the most serious equity thread in a women's health strategy in English history. It matters that the paper exists. It matters more that the women named in this chapter are still, in 2026, waiting for it to mean something in their lives.

Three further women

Let me introduce three more women, because the argument of this chapter lives in them rather than in the statistics, even where the statistics support them.

Etta Mukasa is twenty-four. In the same Refinery29 feature that gave us Natalie, Etta described symptoms that began in her teens and a diagnostic journey that was still ongoing when she spoke (Refinery29, 2025). She had been told, as so many Black British women are, that her pain was within normal range, that she should try hormonal contraception, that she should lose weight. She had not, at the time of the interview, had a laparoscopy. She was not alone; she is one of many young Black British women whose endometriosis will, statistically, not be confirmed until she is in her thirties, by which point the surgical options for fertility preservation have narrowed.

Sophia, also in the Refinery29 feature, is based in the UK. Her story is one of repeated device rejection: her body, over the course of several years, rejected four hormonal coils. "My body kept rejecting the coil. I had it put in like four times, and my body would just knock it back out of place" (Refinery29, 2025).

An endometriosis diagnosis was finally given to her. Her story represents one of those things that are rarely mentioned in the medical literature: the unique problem of seeking treatment when your body has been fighting the illness for several years.

Sam is a Black American woman whose story is documented on the website of the Endometriosis Foundation of America. She has had a history of ninety days of menstruation for five years. She booked three surgeries but cancelled all of them. "That's usually what they like to offer Black women and women of colour," she explained. Several doctors told her that endometriosis is "a white woman's disease" (Endometriosis Foundation of America, cited in Endofound, 2025). I include her here because the pattern is not UK-specific, though the NHS-specific consequences and the NHS-specific remedies obviously are. The fibroid paradox runs on both sides of the Atlantic, and Lupita Nyong'o's advocacy has made it a transatlantic conversation for the first time.

Four women: Natalie, Etta, Sophia, Sam. Each of them was told, in effect, that her body did not come with the right ethnicity for the right disease. Each of them has had her life rearranged around a diagnostic delay that is not, in any clinically defensible sense, a product of random variation in access. It is a product of assumption.

The doctor who said it out loud

I want to give you, in contrast, the voice of a Black British GP who has been willing to name what she sees from inside the system.

Dr Itunu Johnson-Sogbetun is a GP whose writing has, over the past few years, begun to change the British conversation on racism in primary care. In a 2024 essay, she described her own practice. "I have heard other clinicians describe heavy bleeding in Black women as 'normal for African women," she wrote. "I have had to say, more than once, that this is not a clinical description. It is a stereotype. And it is producing preventable harm in my patients" (Johnson-Sogbetun, 2024).

I include Dr Johnson-Sogbetun's voice because I want to be clear that inside the system, many clinicians are actively trying to name and correct exactly the patterns this chapter describes. My experience of training the next generation of midwives at Middlesex University is that the incoming cohort is alert, well-informed, and unwilling to carry forward the inherited patterns of their predecessors. They are trained to notice. They are trained to ask. They are trained to document. They are the reason I have, on balance, some optimism about the decade ahead.

The work, however, is not primarily their work. It is the work of the institutions that employ them: the Royal Colleges that set training standards, the NHS trusts that commission services, the Integrated Care Boards that design pathways, the GP partnerships that run practices. Inside those institutions, the pace of change on racial equity has been glacial. The Renewed Strategy is the most serious attempt at acceleration I have seen. It is still, in the specific lives of the women this chapter names, arriving late.

What we are entitled to expect

I want to end this chapter with what I believe Black British women, South Asian British women, and all ethnic minority women in this country are entitled to expect from the NHS in 2026 and the years following.

They are entitled to consultations in which their description of their own symptoms is treated as clinical evidence, not filtered through a racial presumption about which disease they are likely to have.

They are entitled to referral pathways that do not require the performance of articulate self-advocacy in a second language.

They are entitled to interpretation services that are human, private, and timely, not telephone lines with a family member overhearing.

They are entitled to the same access to fertility preservation, specialist centres, and advanced treatments as white women with comparable clinical presentations.

They are entitled to care from clinicians who have been trained specifically in the ways that cultural and racial assumptions distort clinical reasoning.

They are entitled to be included in research that studies their bodies, rather than being the population in which treatments developed for other bodies are tested after the fact.

They are entitled to a health service that recognises that the 80% of Black women who will develop fibroids by fifty are not a problem to be managed down but a population whose needs are, by any reasonable reading of public health priorities, at the top of the list.

The Renewed Strategy has committed, on paper, to most of these. What the next five years will have to see from Parliament, from the Secretary of State, from the NHS, from the Royal Colleges, from the commissioners, from the clinicians, from the advocates, from the women themselves is for the paper to become reality.

In the next chapter, which is shorter, I want to write about what else has to change to make this possible. Not the structural mechanisms, which this book has been describing throughout, but the culture inside which the structures operate. Because some of what has to change is not strategy. It is a story. And the story is the thing the women in this chapter have been rewriting, one consultation at a time, at great personal cost, for a very long time.

※ ※ ※

CHAPTER EIGHT

Culture, Context, and Care

I want to tell you a story from my own family, because it is the only piece of personal material in this book, and I have thought carefully about including it.

My maternal grandmother grew up in Zimbabwe. She had seven children, several of whom did not survive infancy. She never, in her long life, told any of her daughters or granddaughters anything about the pain she had experienced with her periods, her pregnancies, or her births. Not because she did not have pain. Because, in her generation and her context, the pain was private. It was borne. It was not, by any cultural standard she had been raised with, the kind of thing a woman discussed.

My mother carried some of that with her. While I started my nursing studies, she was quite proud, but she also made sure that I knew I might end up finding myself in professional situations where I was exposed to very private parts that even she would have wished to keep personal. When I started studying midwifery, she made another point which I find interesting even today. She told me that she wished I should always bear in mind that some women, particularly those from specific backgrounds, had spent all their lives not discussing their bodies.

I wish I could say I always understood it. I did not. Early in my career, I asked questions in ways I now realise were culturally inappropriate. I conducted examinations in ways that did not sufficiently account for the fact that the woman in front of me might have had no prior framework for discussing her body with a stranger, let alone a stranger wearing a uniform in a foreign country. I got better. Getting better is the work.

I tell this story because this chapter argues that culture is not a peripheral factor in women's healthcare. It is a central one. And the NHS, which is one of the most multicultural healthcare services in the world, has only in recent years begun to take the implications seriously.

Intergenerational silence

Many women carry, in addition to their own diagnoses, the weight of generations of women before them who were not permitted to speak about theirs.

This is not only a South Asian or African phenomenon, though the specific forms it takes vary culturally. I have met white British women in their sixties whose mothers never discussed menstruation with them, who learned about their periods from a pamphlet at school, and who have, in turn, never discussed their own menstrual health with their daughters. I have met Pakistani women in their thirties for whom the question of endometriosis is complicated by the fact that discussing fertility with an unmarried daughter is, in their family context, taboo. I have met orthodox Jewish women who have navigated mikvah practice and heavy menstrual bleeding with a kind of private ingenuity that the clinical system has not found a way to ask about.

Each of these is a different version of the same fact. Menstrual suffering has, in most cultures, been borne privately and by women alone. The fact that this is now changing, that Lupita Nyong'o can discuss her fibroids on American morning television, that Jen Moore can do a Radio 4 interview about her pain, that Aaliyah's generation is likelier than mine was to be told by teachers that heavy periods are not normal and should be investigated, is the single biggest cultural shift in this territory in my lifetime. It is the reason that some of what this book describes is beginning to be describable in public at all.

For the clinician, the cultural context matters because it shapes what the patient can tell you. A Muslim woman from a conservative family may find it impossible, in a nine-minute appointment with a male GP she does not know, to describe pain during intercourse. A Chinese-British woman whose mother has told her all her life that period pain is karmic may not have the vocabulary to ask whether her pain is abnormal, because the framework of normal-versus-abnormal was not available to her. A Somali woman who has experienced female genital cutting may have specific medical needs that interact with endometriosis in ways her clinician has not been trained to ask about.

The Renewed Strategy's Action 68, launched through the NIHR, is a new funding call focused on how best to improve communication around women's health across the life course, particularly in underserved or marginalised communities (DHSC, 2026, p. 57). This is long-overdue research. It is also a small, welcome sign that the system is beginning to recognise that communication is not a soft skill. It is a clinical infrastructure, and the infrastructure has been underbuilt.

The telephone problem

I want to give you one specific example of how cultural assumptions baked into NHS design can systematically exclude marginalised women.

Telephone consultation has been a common practice since the onset of the pandemic in UK primary care. It is an effective and time-saving method, and it is, for the most part, adequate for dealing with simple medical concerns. It is not adequate for all.

This issue was reflected by Healthwatch Berkshire in their report for 2023 regarding the well-being of women based on a conversation with 580 women. One woman's experience, recorded by Healthwatch Berkshire, was described as follows: "I am very anxious when I talk on the telephone to my doctor because I cannot convey my point clearly; it is much easier if I could speak with them face-to-face." (Healthwatch Berkshire, 2023). Although this woman's name was not disclosed, she was a non-native speaker of English. Her problem did not lie in understanding or processing information. It was phonological. She could convey her point of view face-to-face because a medical practitioner would be able to understand through gestures or physical actions.

The Renewed Strategy's commitment to the analogue-to-digital shift is, on its own terms, positive. Digital infrastructure will benefit many women: those in remote areas, those with caring responsibilities, and those for whom taking half a day off work for an appointment is financially or logistically impossible. It will also, if implemented without care, amplify exactly the exclusion this woman describes. Action 37, committing to Health Store in the NHS App, and Action 38, enhancing and expanding the NHS App as a digital front door, both need to be implemented with deliberate attention to women for whom digital is not neutral (DHSC, 2026, p. 39). The Strategy itself acknowledges this, noting that DHSC will contribute to the government's digital inclusion drive and will make sure in-person appointments remain a choice for all who need and prefer them (DHSC, 2026, p. 39). Whether that principle survives contact with implementation remains to be seen.

Faith, family, and the people who decide

For many women, particularly from South Asian and some African communities, healthcare decisions are not made individually. They are made within family structures in which older women, husbands, and sometimes religious or community leaders play significant roles. This is not, on its own, a problem. It is a cultural reality, and sometimes a source of real support.

It becomes a problem when the clinical system does not know how to work with it. A young British South Asian woman bringing her mother-in-law to an endometriosis consultation may not be doing so because she is dependent. She may be doing so because the mother-in-law is the person in the household who will decide whether she has the surgery being recommended, and a clinician who speaks only to the patient, ignoring the mother-in-law, may find that the surgery does not happen. An older Nigerian woman attending a hysterectomy pre-assessment with her husband is not, in most cases, experiencing coercion. She is attending with the person whose emotional and practical support she needs.

Clinicians, in my experience, often find these dynamics uncomfortable because British medical training, which emphasises patient autonomy, has no strong framework for communal decision-making. The clinician's reflex is to ask to speak to the patient alone. This is not always correct. Sometimes it is. Sometimes, asking a Black British woman whose abusive partner is sitting next to her whether she would like to speak alone is a lifeline. Sometimes, asking a Bangladeshi woman whose supportive husband is translating for her whether she would like to speak alone is an insult. Distinguishing between the two takes cultural competence, and cultural competence takes training that has historically been absent from the medical curriculum.

The Renewed Strategy's Action 35 commits to a new workforce model with core skills, basic, intermediate and advanced that professionals need to deliver high-quality women's healthcare (DHSC, 2026, p.

37). This should include, if it is serious, cultural competence as a core competency rather than an optional extra. Whether it does will become clear in the 10 Year Workforce Plan expected in 2026.

Violence, disclosure, and the consultation room

I want to say something here that is difficult, because it is both common and under-discussed.

A significant minority of women presenting with gynaecological symptoms in British primary care are also experiencing domestic abuse, sexual abuse, or the ongoing consequences of historical trauma. One in eight women in England and Wales in the year ending March 2025 experienced domestic abuse, sexual assault, or stalking (ONS, 2025, cited in DHSC, 2026). The consultation for heavy periods or pelvic pain is sometimes the consultation in which the disclosure could happen, if the clinician knew how to hold the space for it.

The Renewed Strategy's Action 50 commits to a national roll-out of "Steps to Safety", a domestic abuse and sexual violence referral service, with the goal that by 2029 any victim or survivor in England will be able to access help by talking to staff at their general practice (DHSC, 2026, p. 46). Action 53 commits to a new safeguarding learning programme for the entire NHS workforce in 2026, covering all aspects of domestic abuse (DHSC, 2026, p. 47). Action 52 invests up to £50 million in expanding the Child House model for victims of child sexual abuse and exploitation, building on the Lighthouse in Camden (DHSC, 2026, p. 46).

These are concrete commitments. I welcome them. I also note that they will only work if clinicians in general practice are given the time, training, and emotional resources to enact them. A nine-minute consultation is not a disclosure-friendly container. The Strategy's commitments to reducing variation in consultation experience, including through the new GP Patient Survey data quality improvement programme (Action 5), will have to bear on this.

For the woman reading this who is experiencing violence: please know that your gynaecological symptoms may be connected, and that you are entitled to ask your clinician to speak to you alone. The phrase "I'd like to speak to you privately", even if only once during an appointment, is the opening many clinicians are trained to recognise and respond to. If yours does not, that is their failure, not yours.

What cultural competence looks like

I want to end this chapter by describing what good cultural competence actually looks like in a consultation room, because it is sometimes imagined as an elaborate ritual, and it is, in fact, relatively simple.

It looks like a clinician who asks, early in the first consultation, how the patient prefers to be addressed, in what language, and whether there is anyone she would like to be present.

It looks like a clinician who does not assume, based on the patient's name or appearance, what her religious or cultural practices are, but who asks about practices that may be clinically relevant, modesty preferences during examination, fasting that may affect a procedure, and dietary factors that may affect a medication.

It looks like a clinician who does not leap to diagnose "normal for African women" when a Black woman describes heavy bleeding, and who does not leap to diagnose "stress" when a South Asian woman describes pelvic pain, and who does not leap to any conclusion from a patient's demographic rather than her presentation.

It looks like a clinician who recognises that interpretation by a family member is not always appropriate, and who knows how to access the NHS interpreting service, which exists in every trust and is free.

It looks like a clinician who knows that the woman in front of her may have been trained for her whole life not to discuss her body with strangers, and who creates, within the nine minutes available, a small space in which the discussion can happen.

And it looks like a clinician who, at the end of the appointment, says a version of: "I believe you, I have taken this seriously, and this is what happens next." This sentence, in my experience, is the single most therapeutic sentence a clinician can offer. It is seldom said. When it is, women remember it for decades.

The structural work of the Renewed Strategy will take years. The therapeutic sentence lasts for four seconds. Both are not competing with the other. Both are equally important. The subsequent sections in this book will focus on the concept of better treatment and how we can achieve it.

PART V

Better Care Is Possible

CHAPTER NINE

What Better Care Looks Like

I have spent the last eight chapters telling you, in some detail, what has been going wrong. I want to spend this one telling you what right looks like.

I will do this in two ways. First, I will describe care as I have seen it delivered, in real rooms, in real NHS trusts, in real countries around the world, when the architecture supports it. Some of what I am about to describe exists already in the UK, in pockets. Some of it exists in other health systems. None of it is science fiction.

Second, I will map that description against the commitments the Renewed Women's Health Strategy has now made. This is the test the Strategy has set itself. Either the commitments are delivered, and the picture below becomes the norm in the lifetime of the current Parliament, or they are not delivered, and the next government's strategy will read, in ten years, very much like this one.

I have no patience left for another round of the same document. I hope you do not either.

The first visit

Imagine a woman, let us say Aaliyah, grown older, now nineteen, walking into her GP's surgery in 2030.

She has been having heavy, painful periods for five years. She has missed school on thirty-six days during her GCSEs and A levels. She has begun to recognise that what she experiences is not what her friends experience. She books an appointment. The receptionist, instead of asking what it is about, uses a digital triage system that asks a few targeted questions and books her into a longer, twenty-minute gynaecology-flagged appointment with a clinician who has women's health as a specialist interest. This clinician may be a GP, a nurse practitioner, or an advanced practitioner within a neighbourhood women's health service because under the Renewed Strategy's commitment to neighbourhood-based care, the single point of access now directs women to the right professional, not just the nearest one (DHSC, 2026, Actions 28–30).

Aaliyah arrives with a symptom tracker she has kept for three months, not because she had to research how to make one, but because the NHS App reminded her to, and the tracker is integrated into her patient record (DHSC, 2026, Action 38). The clinician reviews the data in the first minute. She asks Aaliyah about the impact on school, on sleep, on her mood, and she writes it down. She examines her, consensually, with Aaliyah's full understanding of what is happening and why. She explains that the symptoms Aaliyah describes are consistent with several possible conditions, including endometriosis, fibroids, and adenomyosis, and that the next step is investigation, not further reassurance.

She refers Aaliyah, that day, to the neighbourhood women's health service for imaging and specialist assessment. The referral is tracked in the NHS App. Aaliyah has a scan within six weeks. The scan suggests fibroids, but not the whole picture. A specialist endometriosis assessment follows. Within four months of her first appointment, Aaliyah has a confirmed diagnosis, a shared decision-making conversation about her treatment options, and a clear care plan.

This is not a fantasy. It is what the Strategy, if delivered, has promised her.

The integrated pathway

The most significant structural commitment in the Renewed Strategy is the single point of access for gynaecology referrals (Action 28), which will direct women rather than requiring them to navigate separate services to the right place at the right time. Combined with Action 29, which commits to standardised clinical pathways for heavy periods, menopause and uro-gynaecology within three years, this represents a genuine restructuring of the first stage of care (DHSC, 2026, p. 36).

What will this feel like for a woman? It means that the GP who suspects endometriosis does not refer her to a general gynaecology clinic that then re-refers her to a specialist. The single point of access triages her directly. It means that the woman with heavy periods does not have four separate appointments at four different sites for her consultation, her scan, her biopsy and her treatment. The standardised pathway combines them.

It also means, crucially, that the information moves with the patient. One of the most demoralising features of current care is the requirement to repeat your story to every new professional because the previous professional's notes have not arrived. The NHS App's Single Patient Record, due in 2028, is intended to fix this. Every clinician the woman sees will access the same record, see the same history, and not require her to reconstruct it from memory (DHSC, 2026, p. 39).

These are not small things. They strip out all the invisible labour required from women to manage their own healthcare arrangements. Instead, they place this burden back where it belongs – within the system.

The community models

What I would like to do here is illustrate for you the actual appearance of a neighbourhood-based women's health clinic.

The Sunderland Women's Health Hub in the Pallion Health Centre, North East England, has been up and running as a pilot scheme since 2023. It brings together, in a single community-based location, GP services with specialist women's health training, advanced practitioners, nurses, and sonographers. It provides LARC fitting, cervical screening support, menopause assessment, ultrasonography, phlebotomy, and outreach clinics at women's refuges and other community sites. Women played a central role in its co-design (DHSC, 2026, p. 38).

The results: improved timely access, reduced unnecessary hospital referrals, and increased uptake of women's health services, particularly among underserved groups. An independent evaluation by the NIHR Applied Research Collaboration North East and North Cumbria found that for every £1 invested, the hub generates £8 in benefits over ten years (DHSC, 2026, p. 38).

Similar models exist in Cheshire and Merseyside, where a pilot across nine local areas is expanding LARC access for all clinical indications. Two areas have already committed to recurrent provision, and seven of nine Places are projected to offer LARC for all indications by late 2026 (DHSC, 2026, p. 25). In Dorset, a women's health programme has created an online resource hub, uploaded five digital apps to the Our Dorset ORCHA library, and achieved 28,868 views of its online health resources (DHSC, 2026, p. 83).

These are not pilots any more. They are working models. The question facing the Strategy is whether the commitment to a regional specialist centre in every NHS region (Action 30) and to neighbourhood women's health services across England (Action 35) will be funded at the scale required for every woman to reach one without an hour's drive.

Digital, done well

The Renewed Strategy commits to NHS Online, a virtual hospital, with menstrual problems and menopause among the first nine pathways established, launching in 2027 (Action 36). It also commits to the NHS App as a digital front door, including appointment booking, record access, advice, and care plan management (Action 38).

Done well, digital transforms women's access to care. It allows a woman in a remote area to consult a specialist without a day's travel. It allows a working woman to book appointments outside office hours. It allows a woman with caring responsibilities to attend appointments from home. It gives women access to their own records, which, in my clinical experience, is one of the most empowering interventions possible.

Done badly, digital exacerbates inequality. The woman who does not speak English as a first language, who does not have a smartphone, and who cannot read comfortably on a screen is left further behind. The Strategy acknowledges this, the DHSC commits to the government's digital inclusion drive and to keeping in-person appointments available for all who need and prefer them (DHSC, 2026, p. 39). Whether this holds in practice will be tested by the women least able to articulate their exclusion.

I want to flag one specific commitment that seems to me to have unusual potential. Action 6 is the launch of My Choices in the NHS App, enabling people to find and compare providers on measures including waiting times, outcomes, and patient experience (DHSC, 2026, p. 21). If implemented with genuine transparency, this would give women something they have not had in the NHS before: real-time comparative information about where to seek care. It would also create genuine pressure on under-performing services, because women who can choose will move, and services will have to improve to retain them.

Equity caveat applies here as well. A woman with access to technology, time, and confidence will be able to use My Choices. Without these resources, she will not. This tool is valuable, but it should not be the only means by which women receive better care.

Research that involves us

One of the key structural considerations of the Strategy is research. Women have historically been under-represented in clinical trials, leading to drug dosages calibrated for male bodies, diagnostic criteria that miss how conditions present in women, and treatment protocols that do not account for female biology (Criado Perez, 2019).

The Strategy's Action 103 commits that NIHR will only fund research that appropriately considers sex-based differences, meaning that research which should but does not take account of sex-based differences will no longer receive public funding (DHSC, 2026, p. 79). This is a significant shift in the funding architecture. Combined with Action 108, which integrates the Be Part of Research service into the NHS App and commits to matching patients automatically with studies based on their own health data, it begins to rebuild the research base on which evidence-based medicine for women depends.

Action 115 commits to a new accelerator for female founders with innovations addressing women's health priorities. FemTech women's health technology has historically received only 4 to 5% of digital health investment globally, a figure the Strategy rightly treats as evidence that the market has been failing this territory (DHSC, 2026, p. 79, citing Sheffield Olympic Legacy Park). Directed public investment to correct this, combined with the new FemTech healthcare challenge (Action 111) with £1.5 million to support systems working with promising developers, is a small but structurally important signal.

I want to be honest about the gap between research commitment and research delivery. The NIHR has funded important research on endometriosis and fibroids in recent years, but the cumulative investment in these conditions remains a fraction of what has been invested in comparable conditions that affect men more equally. Closing that gap will take years. It will also require the voices of women with these conditions to be embedded in the research agenda itself. The Strategy's co-production commitments are welcome; whether they translate into research questions that women themselves would ask remains to be seen.

Accountability

The most innovative commitment in the Strategy, to my eye, is Action 4: patient power payments. This would vary the amount NHS trusts are reimbursed, depending on women's feedback on their experiences, particularly around pain management. Gynaecology services are prioritised as the first test (DHSC, 2026, p. 21).

This is genuinely novel. It creates the first structural financial incentive in the NHS for trusts to listen to women. A trust that consistently delivers poor experiences, including inadequate pain management for hysteroscopy, is still running at one in three women reporting severe pain, and reimbursement would be withheld and redirected to improving those services.

Combined with Action 2 (a new National Director of Patient Experience, appointed from this year) and Action 32 (a publicly available women's health data dashboard providing neighbourhood-level comparable data), the Strategy has begun to build an accountability architecture that does not currently exist (DHSC, 2026, pp. 20, 36).

I have been in many meetings over the years where NHS performance on women's health was discussed in aggregate, in private, and with no mechanism for consequence. What the Strategy commits to is different. Performance will be published, comparable, and tied to payment. This is the kind of structural accountability that changes behaviour when everything else has failed. Whether it is delivered will determine whether the Strategy becomes the document that turned the tide or the document that promised to.

Jess's Rule, Martha's Rule, and the new culture of listening

I want to highlight two reforms already in place that are worth understanding.

Jess's Rule is named for Jessica Brady, who died from cancer after her condition was missed or dismissed despite more than twenty GP appointments (DHSC, 2026, p. 2). It requires GP teams to "reflect, review, and rethink" when a patient presents three times with the same or escalating symptoms. In effect, three appointments without a diagnosis are a trigger for a different kind of conversation.

Martha's Rule, rolled out to every acute hospital in England, allows patients, families and carers to escalate concerns for review by a different clinical team if they believe someone is deteriorating and not being listened to (DHSC, 2026, pp. 20–21). This is now standard across English acute care.

Both rules came from the deaths of women and girls whose concerns were not heeded. Both are, in my view, structurally significant. They do not solve medical misogyny. They do create documented pressure points at which the system is required to pause and listen. If a woman with endometriosis has been to her GP three times, Jess's Rule now applies. She is entitled to invoke it. Many women do not know this. Knowing it is itself a form of power.

What has to be true for this to work

I want to end this chapter by being direct about the conditions under which the Strategy's vision will actually be delivered.

First, sustained funding. The Strategy commits substantial sums of £200 million for Healthy Babies, £50 million for child sexual abuse and exploitation services, £2.6 million for DEXA scanners, £1.5 million for the FemTech challenge, and various smaller pots, but these are not large in the context of NHS spend as a whole. The test will be whether commitments survive the Treasury's attention over a decade of implementation.

Second, the workforce. The promised expansion of neighbourhood women's health services requires clinicians. The 10 Year Workforce Plan, due for publication this year, will have to commit not only to training new midwives, GPs with women's health interests, and advanced practitioners, but also to retaining the staff we already have. NHS staff retention in women's health specialities has been a concern for years.

Third, accountability. The dashboard, the PREMs, the patient power payments, and the National Director of Patient Experience: all of these only matter if the data they produce is actually acted on. The Strategy commits to transparency. What it has not yet committed to is the consequence structure for trusts that consistently fail beyond the financial reimbursement mechanism, which applies only to specific pathways initially.

Fourth, the voices that are supposed to be partners. The Women's Voices Partnership is a good idea. It will only work if it genuinely includes organisations representing the most marginalised women, and if its input is binding rather than decorative. This is the test that has failed in previous iterations of patient voice in the NHS.

Fifth, and most importantly, honesty. The Strategy is the most honest government document I have seen on women's health. Its acknowledgements of sexism, medical misogyny, systemic failure, and racial inequality are on the public record. That honesty has to carry through every stage of implementation. It cannot now be retreated from. The women who live with these conditions will not let it be.

The next chapter is about the women who have been doing the work of building what the state has, until now, not been willing to build. It is the chapter of which I am proudest to be part.

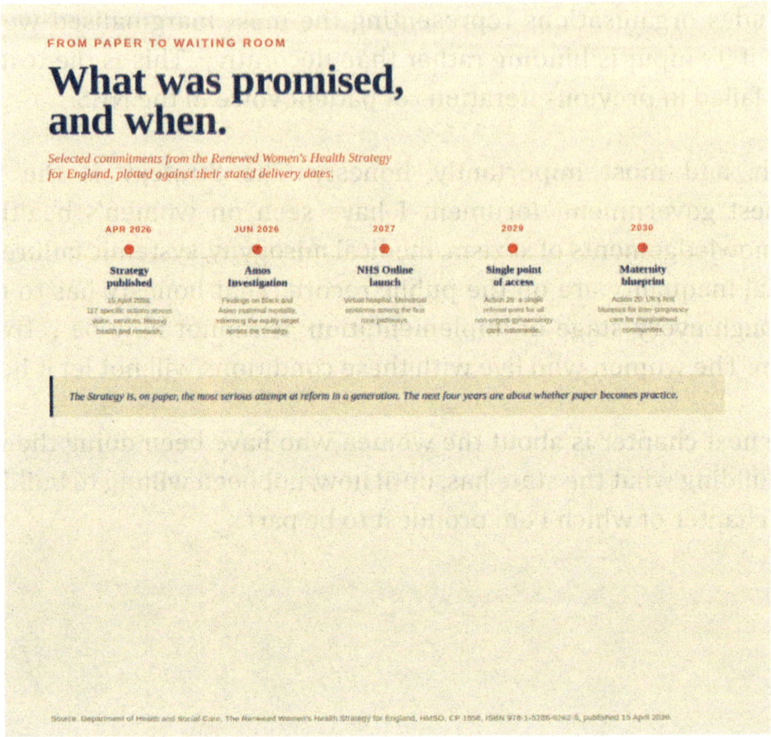

Figure 12. The Renewed Women's Health Strategy: what was promised, and when.

※ ※ ※

CHAPTER TEN

Community, Knowledge, and Support

Emma Cox has been the chief executive of Endometriosis UK since 2018. In that time, her charity has become the single most important civil society voice for British women with this disease. It has produced the survey data that this book, the Renewed Women's Health Strategy, and the House of Commons' March 2026 debate have all cited. It has trained clinicians, advised MPs, written guidance, and, on its helpline, answered the phone to tens of thousands of women who did not know, before they rang, that anyone would believe them.

I want to begin this chapter with Endometriosis UK because I want to make a claim that I will defend over the next fifteen or so pages. Civil society charities, community organisations, online networks, and small advocacy groups have been doing the work for which the state refused to take responsibility. The Strategy now promises the state will begin to do some of that work itself. It is essential to understand what the community has done, and continues to do, because without it, there is no movement and without movement, there is no Strategy.

This chapter is also the one in which I disclose, in some detail, my own role as the founder of Vina, the women's health platform. I want to handle that disclosure honestly rather than quietly, so I am placing it in the middle of this chapter. Vina is one of many organisations in the ecosystem I am describing. It is not the most important. It exists because the ecosystem has not been enough and because I, like the founders of the other organisations, saw a gap I could personally try to fill. The rest of this chapter belongs to the organisations that have been doing this work far longer than I have.

The charities that have held the line

Endometriosis UK was founded in 1981. It has run, continuously, through four decades of medical neglect and policy silence. It runs a national helpline, regional support groups, a menstrual wellbeing schools programme, professional education for clinicians, and a campaigning arm that has shaped UK policy. Its 2024 survey of more than 4,300 diagnosed women is the largest picture of the British diagnostic experience we have (Endometriosis UK, 2024). Emma Cox's voice is quoted in almost every serious piece of British journalism on endometriosis, and for good reason: she has done the work.

Cysters was founded by Neelam Heera-Shergill in Birmingham in 2015. It began as a community support group for South Asian women with reproductive and mental health conditions, and grew into a national charity serving Black and minority ethnic women across the UK. Heera-Shergill has been willing to say, repeatedly and on the record, what many others have not: that the failures of UK reproductive healthcare fall disproportionately on Black and Asian women, and that cultural competence is not an optional extra. Her organisation produces research, runs support groups, and has become a key consultee for policy-makers. The Renewed Strategy's Women's Voices Partnership will almost certainly include Cysters; it would be an insult to the evidence base if it did not (RCOG, 2026).

The Adeno Gang, founded by Tanya Simon-Hall, is the UK's principal advocacy network for women with adenomyosis. Adenomyosis, the growth of endometrial tissue into the muscular wall of the uterus, has been historically even more under-recognised than endometriosis, partly because it was widely thought to be diagnosable only at hysterectomy. Simon-Hall's network has forced the condition into public awareness, pushed for its inclusion in clinical guidelines, and given women who had not previously had a community a place to find one.

The Fibroid Network focuses specifically on women with uterine fibroids, with particular attention to the disproportionate burden on Black women. Wellbeing of Women, founded in 1964 as the Childbirth Research Centre, funds UK research on women's reproductive health and has published some of the most influential British reports on menstrual disease, including the 2025 "Just a Period" report that this book cites repeatedly (Wellbeing of Women, 2025).

Black Womxn's Health, Five X More, and Jamii are among the organisations focused specifically on Black women's health in the UK, across reproductive, maternal, and mental health domains. Their work, and the voices within them, have begun to shift what the NHS can be expected to acknowledge about race and care.

These are not fringe organisations. For a large number of women suffering from such diseases in Britain, they act as the main source of knowledge, care, and representation. They do the work that the NHS did not. The Renewed Strategy acknowledges their existence and commits, via the Women's Voices Partnership, to bring them formally into policy-making (DHSC, 2026, Action 1). This is a recognition long overdue.

The online communities

Outside the registered charities, there is a vast and largely invisible infrastructure of online communities that has transformed what it feels like to live with endometriosis, fibroids and adenomyosis in the UK.

Facebook groups are the backbone of much of this. Closed groups with thousands of members exist for each condition, for women in particular regions of the UK, for women of specific ethnic backgrounds, and for women at specific stages of the diagnostic journey. They are moderated, usually by volunteers, often by women whose own diagnoses are years old. They are the place where a newly diagnosed woman finds out what questions to ask at her next appointment, which consultants in her area are known to be good, and what the realistic recovery time is for a laparoscopy at the trust she has been referred to.

These two social media platforms operate in different ways. The subreddit communities on Reddit dedicated to endometriosis, fibroids, and adenomyosis are mostly text-driven and anonymous, attracting women who post information based on their experiences. However, TikTok has increasingly become the go-to social media platform for women who need information on these topics. In this context, the efforts made by Dr Karen Tang through her TikTok account @ KarenTangMD, who creates short, evidence-based videos that discuss menstruation and pelvic pain issues, have had more influence than all government campaigns ever created (Tang, 2024).

It would be unfair to paint the online community in one brushstroke only. It should be noted that the online world is also the source of many misconceptions; some of them are even deliberately spread for financial benefit by companies offering wellness products. The idea that endometriosis can be reversed by following certain dietary recommendations is a popular example of such a misconception, which lacks a scientific basis altogether. Women who look for answers online should be critical, yet it is difficult for them due to the nature of the internet space.

Nonetheless, the overall impact has been highly positive. While in 2005 she would have endured her pain alone, in isolation, and thinking it was something to be ashamed of because it was only happening to her, in 2026, she will probably know there are other women like her. There is a culture change, even though the medical one is lagging.

What I've made, and why

Next, the disclosure I have made both here and in my Author's Note. I am the co-founder of Vina, the UK women's health app. What follows is an attempt at describing Vina as accurately as possible without any marketing spin.

Vina was created out of years spent observing within the NHS, seeing certain trends play out time and time again and noticing the same women slipping through the cracks each time. I watched midwives trying to support women through heavy, complex gynaecological histories and having neither the time nor the integrated information to do it well. I watched the women themselves piecing together their own care from charities, online communities, GP appointments they had to fight for, and private care they could not always afford. I watched Black British women in particular receive systematically worse care, from a system that was supposed to treat them equally, and I watched the research community take years to catch up with what was already obvious in the clinic.

Vina is a platform designed to give women an integrated space for tracking, information, community, and, in partnership with the NHS and private providers, care coordination. It is not a replacement for the NHS. It is not, despite what some competitor platforms market themselves as, a cure or a treatment. It is an attempt to put into one place the tools that women were having to assemble from fourteen different sources, and to do so in a way that is specifically designed around the experiences of Black and ethnically diverse British women, because those are the women I know best and those are the women most poorly served by the existing landscape.

Vina makes me proud, but I am also realistic about its limitations. It is one tool among others. It does not have the capacity to address the underlying structural issues presented in this book. It cannot, in itself, make the queue for gynaecological services shorter or eradicate medical misogyny. But what it can do is minimise the invisible work women need to do to organise their own treatment, and it can offer women who have not found support elsewhere a reliable resource.

I am telling you this so that you, as the reader, will know this and evaluate my arguments accordingly. I have not hidden the connection, and I have not used this book as a marketing vehicle. If you are interested in Vina, you will find it. If you are not, nothing in this book requires you to engage with it. The ecosystem I have described above exists independently of Vina, and much of it predates Vina by decades. Those organisations, not mine, are the ones that have held the line longest. They deserve the attention.

The power of naming

I want to return to something I said in the first chapter. The reassurance trap works because it is not named. Once named, it begins to lose its power.

The same principle applies to much of what this book describes. Medical misogyny is now named in a government document. Racial disparity in maternal mortality is named in government commitments to close the gap. The fibroid paradox, the statistical and presumptive pattern by which Black women are assumed to have fibroids, not endometriosis, regardless of their presentation, is now described, if not yet fully addressed. The emotional cost of self-advocacy is named in research and in patient testimony. The telephone problem, the continuity problem, the fragmentation problem: all of these now have names.

Naming is not solving. But naming is the first step. Things that cannot be described cannot be addressed. Things that can be described can, at least in principle, be changed.

The community organisations in this chapter have been the primary names. They have been the ones saying, for years, what the state has only recently been willing to say. The Strategy's language has the voices of Emma Cox, Neelam Heera-Shergill, Tanya Simon-Hall, Dr Itunu Johnson-Sogbetun and their peers woven through it, whether or not the Strategy attributes the language to them. They have done the translation work that turned women's private suffering into public policy. They are the reason this book can exist at all.

What a woman can do today

I want to end this chapter with something practical, because community is not only an abstract support. It is something you can use this afternoon.

If you are reading this and you do not know where to start, Endometriosis UK's helpline is 0808 808 2227. It is free to call, staffed by trained volunteers, and available from Monday to Friday during daytime hours. The charity's website has a symptom checker, a directory of local support groups, and resources you can download to prepare for appointments. Wellbeing of Women and Cysters have similar resources. Appendix E provides information about the important UK organisations and their contact details.

If you want to look up some kind of online community, then I would recommend looking into joining a private Facebook page devoted to your specific illness and your local area. Such private groups usually have much better moderation than public pages on Reddit and Twitter. TikTok can help discover resources, but should not be used as a reliable medical tool by any means.

If you just got diagnosed, then there is no need for you to handle your treatment entirely alone. The charities will help you to get ready for your consultation with the specialist, learn your medical options, and determine when you should question some of the recommendations. Furthermore, the charities can help you connect with women who have gone through a similar process of getting their diagnosis if you so desire.

Aspiring advocates can rest assured that the organisations mentioned in this chapter are all actively recruiting volunteers. Opportunities span from helplines to social media campaigning to legislative advocacy. Training will be provided by the organisations themselves, as they require your help.

Finally, should you have any material to contribute towards their funding, please do so. Civil society has had the funding of these organisations down to its last dollar due to decades of neglect. It is only now that the Renewed Strategy begins to provide government funding for them.

The next hundred years

But before I end this chapter, I want to comment on the subject of time.

The National Health Service was established in 1948. The next fifty years after that were devoted to women's reproductive health being an afterthought inadequately funded and studied, at best. Then, for the following twenty years, there were initial discussions regarding it.

Now, in the final five years, it has become an integral part of political discourse, something which could hardly have been imagined at the start of my career.

It did not occur this way simply because some governmental decision was made for it to occur. It happened because women decided, collectively in the millions, that they would no longer remain silent about their plight. This was made possible by Jen Moore, Hayley and Sarah Beaton, Natalie, Lupita Nyong'o, and countless other women who spoke out about their experiences. It happened because of Emma Cox, Neelam Heera-Shergill, and so many others who created the organisations that got us this far.

It is, in that way, a result of civil society pressures which have finally passed a certain boundary line. It is not the end of the narrative. It is only the first time that governments have admitted to a long tale which had already been going on. The next hundred years of British women's healthcare will be shaped by what happens next. By whether the Strategy's commitments are delivered. Whether the women's voices that have produced the pressure continue to be heard once they are formally invited into policy-making. Whether the money follows the words. Whether the women who come after Aaliyah, the girls entering adolescence now, the children not yet born, inherit a system fundamentally different from the one that failed their mothers and grandmothers.

This is not, I want to be clear, a hope I am expressing as an outsider. It is the work I have spent my career on, and it is work I intend to continue. The book you have nearly finished is part of it. The Patient Manifesto that follows is part of it. The organisations listed in the Appendix are part of it. The conversations you have with your GP, your MP, your partner, your daughter, your colleague, are part of it.

All of this is part of it. You are part of it.

Thank you for reading.

CONCLUSION

Moving Forward

On the 5th of March 2026, in the House of Commons, an MP rose to describe what women with endometriosis and fibroids had been enduring for decades. She used the words "shameful delays". She named the statistic that twenty MPs currently in the House would, on simple probability, be living with endometriosis themselves. She quoted patients by name. She asked the government to act.

Six weeks later, the Renewed Women's Health Strategy for England was published. A government department that had previously taken years to acknowledge the simplest facts of women's reproductive health had written, in its Secretary of State's signed foreword, the phrase "an appalling culture of medical misogyny" (DHSC, 2026, p. 2). The same document is committed to one hundred and seventeen specific actions across voice, services, lifelong health, and research.

I want to be honest at the end of this book about what I believe and what I do not believe.

I believe the Strategy is the most serious government response to women's health in my professional lifetime. It names what needed naming. It commits funds, however modestly. It creates accountability structures that did not previously exist. Its equity thread, if delivered, would begin to close the gap that has killed and hospitalised Black and ethnic minority women disproportionately for generations.

I do not believe, and I want to be clear about this, that the Strategy on its own will deliver. Paper is the cheapest substance in Whitehall. I have seen promises like this before. I watched, between 2022 and 2025, the previous Women's Health Strategy under a different government fail to translate into meaningful improvements in access, experience, or outcomes, a failure that the current Strategy itself acknowledges in its opening pages (DHSC, 2026, p. 9). What is different this time is the acknowledgement of why the previous strategy failed, and the commitment to restructure rather than to incrementally improve. What is not yet different is delivery. Delivery is the test.

What the fight requires now

I want to set out, plainly, what I believe has to happen for the Strategy to become the document that turned the tide on women's healthcare in this country.

NICE, the National Institute for Health and Care Excellence, must implement the updated endometriosis guideline with binding force.

This requirement for a specialist referral after three months was specified by NICE in its 2024 guidelines. Unfortunately, it is not consistently observed. This needs to be monitored and enforced.

NHS England should be compelled to provide the single-entry point for gynaecology referrals by the specified deadline, and the budget allocated to this should be adequate for every neighbourhood in England, not only the test ones. The waiting list for gynaecology should be reduced, not to the eighteen-week standard but below this as a lower limit, and the women with the longest wait times need to be reported.

GP training needs to be revamped. All GP trainees in the UK need to undergo mandatory, examinable training in endometriosis, fibroids, adenomyosis, and racial biases in pain assessment before they graduate. This is entirely possible via the power held by the Royal College of General Practitioners and the GMC.

There needs to be a publication annually from the Royal Colleges of RCOG, RCM, RCGP, and RCN on women's health outcomes per trust, per region, and per ethnicity. Professional accountability alone will not solve anything; it has failed to work until now.

Commitment to action needs naming ministers when commitments are missed. The National Director of Patient Experience, who is committed to doing this, should publish quarterly reports on the status of actions in the Strategy of 117 commitments, listing the minister responsible for each one.

The Women's Voices Partnership must include, from its establishment, the advocacy organisations and individual women most disadvantaged by the current system. Its input must be binding, not advisory. A partnership that does not change what is decided is not a partnership. It is a theatre.

Research funding must shift proportionately. The NIHR commitment that research failing to consider sex-based differences will no longer be funded is a start. It must be matched by a commitment to invest in women's reproductive health research at a level proportionate to its population impact.

And above all, the women must continue to speak. The Strategy exists because they did. Its delivery will depend on them continuing to.

What a reader can do this week

I want to end with actions, because every call for collective change has to translate into individual action, or it evaporates.

If you are a woman reading this with symptoms that have been dismissed, your next GP appointment is an opportunity. Bring the tracker from Appendix B. Ask the question from Appendix A: "If it isn't endometriosis or fibroids, what else could this be, and what investigation would rule it out?" If you are refused investigation, ask for the refusal to be documented. If you are still refused, request a second opinion or a referral from a different GP in your practice. You do not need permission to do this.

If you are reading this and a woman you love is struggling, go with her to her appointment. Believe her out loud. Say, in the room, that you have watched her be in pain for six months, and you are concerned it is not being investigated. The architecture of the consultation is not fair; use whatever leverage you have.

If you are reading this and you are well, or whose own care has been adequate, write to your MP. The Strategy is only as strong as the political pressure sustaining it. Write and say you have read this book, you have understood what women in your constituency are experiencing, and you expect your MP to track the delivery of the 117 actions. Mention Jen Moore, Hayley, Sarah Beaton, Natalie, and Lupita Nyong'o. Names matter. So do constituents who notice.

If you are a clinician reading this, you know already what you can do. You can listen to the next woman who sits in front of you as if she might be right. You can cite NICE 2024 when a colleague normalises heavy periods. You can ask, in your team meetings, how your referral patterns break down by ethnicity. You can advocate, where you can, for the structural changes the Strategy promises. You are not the problem. But you are inside the architecture, and the architecture needs clinicians willing to notice.

If you are a policy-maker, you have the Strategy in front of you. Deliver it. Do not let it become another document that promised. Deliver it.

If you are an employer or an HR lead, read the Employment Rights Act 2025 obligations carefully. The new requirement, coming in 2027, for employers of 250 or more staff to publish action plans including menopause support, means that planning starts now. Women at your organisation will benefit. So will your retention rates.

And if you have the resources to donate to Endometriosis UK, Wellbeing of Women, Cysters, Black Womxn's Health, the Adeno Gang, the Fibroid Network, or any of the organisations listed in Appendix E: please do. They carried the load for decades. They will carry it for years to come.

The last story

I began this book with Aaliyah, the fourteen-year-old who asked me whether this was going to be her whole life now.

I want to end with her, because a book like this should finish in a real room with a real woman, not in abstraction.

When I spoke to Aaliyah's mother six months after that first conversation, Aaliyah had been referred to a gynaecologist. A scan had been ordered. The possibility of endometriosis as a tentative diagnosis had come up for the first time. She was not healed. She continued to be absent from school, although not for as many days as she had been. She was still experiencing pain, but it had gained a name and, by doing so, altered the way she experienced it.

"She's not ashamed anymore," her mother explained in one of my favourite quotes. "She used to hide it all. Now she tells her friends and says, 'I have got endometriosis. It's a condition. They're treating me for it.'"

This is it, right here, this move, in essence. From personal shame to owned condition. From the girl who had to wonder if this would always be her life to the girl who knows that this will never be her body again and that the fight is hers to participate in.

She won't have to go through the same struggles that her grandmother went through. She won't go through anything that I had to. She will have, if everything we've talked about in the Strategy happens, a life where the thought of "Could this be endometriosis?" isn't raised during her tenth doctor's appointment, but during her first, by a doctor who knows to look for it. Going through the process of referral doesn't mean having to become an expert on the issue yourself. Having brown skin doesn't mean you're automatically ruled out for a certain diagnosis. Where pain is investigated, not ignored.

This is the battle. And this is just the start.

I want to thank all the women who were involved in helping name this struggle. I want to thank the readers who got to this point. And I am determined to keep going forward from here.

Sarah Chitongo

London, April 2026

The Patient Manifesto

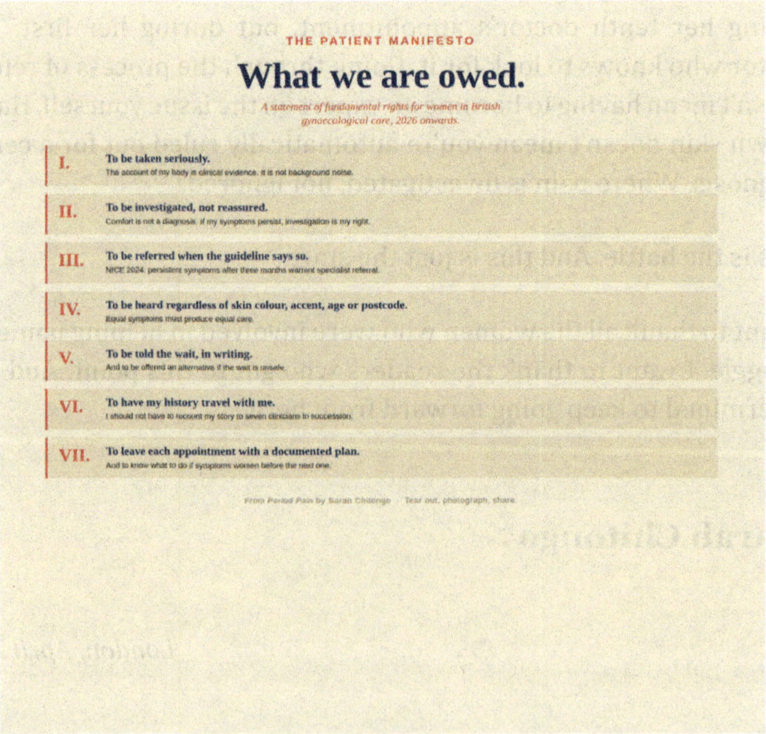

Figure 13. The Patient Manifesto.

Appendix A: The Appointment Script

This appendix contains a set of scripted questions and sentences you can use in GP consultations to move a conversation from reassurance to investigation. None of these is aggressive. All of them are clinical. They have been drafted in discussion with women who had their own diagnoses expedited due to employing such terminology.

Before your appointment

Jot down the following on one sheet of paper:

- The date you first noticed your symptoms, and how they have progressed.
- Your pain score over the past two menstrual cycles, measured from zero to ten on average.
- The effect on your day-to-day life: days lost at work or school, problems with sexual activity, insomnia, social relations, and mood swings.

- Anything you have attempted yourself (drugs, nutrition, birth control), and whether anything worked for you.

- Family history of endometriosis, uterine fibroids, adenomyosis, or reproductive cancers.

Opening statement during appointment

"I have documented my symptoms over the past two months. Perhaps I could share this information with you to analyse the trend."

This shift in tone turns the appointment into a more analytical process than just complaint-making.

The core questions

"If it isn't endometriosis or fibroids, what else could this be, and what investigation would rule it out?"

This question forces differential diagnosis, which is the clinical mode GPs are best at. It is very difficult for a GP to respond with reassurance to this question without making the refusal explicit.

If the investigation is refused

"Could you document in my notes today that I asked for an investigation and was advised against it?"

This sentence converts an informal encounter into a documented one. Most GPs, faced with writing this down, will reconsider.

If the refusal persists

"What are your reasons for not referring me at this point, in terms of the NICE guideline on endometriosis or fibroids?"

The NICE guideline on endometriosis (NG73, updated 2024) recommends specialist referral when symptoms persist despite management for three months. Your GP should be able to explain why the guideline does not apply to you. If they cannot, you have the right to a second opinion.

Asking for a second opinion

"I'd like to request a second opinion within the practice. Could I be booked with a different GP, ideally one with a special interest in women's health?"

You do not need to justify this request. The NHS constitution guarantees your right to a second opinion.

Asking for a specialist referral

"Given my symptoms have persisted despite three months of management, I'd like to be referred to a gynaecologist for specialist assessment."

If the response is that the waiting list is long, you can follow up with: "I understand the wait may be long. I'd still like to be on the list from today."

If you are a Black woman and suspect bias

"I'm aware that endometriosis has historically been underdiagnosed in Black women. I'd like to make sure we're considering it in my differential, not just ruling it out based on statistical assumptions."

This sentence names the fibroid paradox without accusing your GP of bias. Most will respond by ordering an appropriate investigation.

For fertility concerns

"I'm concerned about the impact of this condition on my fertility. Could we discuss referral for fertility assessment alongside investigation of the underlying condition?"

Before you leave the appointment

"Could I please have a summary of today's plan what has been agreed, what tests will be ordered, when I'll hear back, and what I should do if symptoms worsen in the meantime?"

This is your right. It prevents the informal appointment from becoming an unactioned one.

Appendix B: The Symptom Tracker

A printable template for tracking your symptoms across one full cycle. Complete each evening. Takes under two minutes per day. Bring to every GP and specialist appointment.

What to track each day

- Date and cycle day (day 1 = first day of period)
- Bleeding: none / light / moderate / heavy / flooding
- Pain score, 0–10 (0 = none, 10 = worst imaginable)
- Location of pain: pelvic, lower back, legs, bowel, bladder, chest, other
- Bowel symptoms: normal / constipated / diarrhoea / painful bowel movements
- Bladder symptoms: normal / urgent / frequent / painful
- Fatigue, 0–10

- Mood, in one word

- Impact: Did pain or bleeding affect work, sex, sleep, exercise, or socialising today?

- Medication taken and dose

What this produces

After 28 days, you will have a document showing:

- How many days of your cycle involve pain scores of 7 or higher

- Whether bowel and bladder symptoms correlate with your cycle

- How many days have you missed work, school, or key activities

- Whether the medication you have tried is actually working

- A pattern, in data, that any clinician can read in thirty seconds

How to present it

Print two copies: one for the clinician, one for your own records. Hand the clinician's copy over in the first minute of your appointment. Do not apologise for bringing it. Say: "This is my symptom record for the last month. I'd like us to look at the pattern together."

Appendix C: Red Flag Checklist

These are symptoms that should never be reassured away without investigation. If you are experiencing any of them, they warrant urgent referral under current NICE guidelines.

Pain

- Pain that prevents you from attending work, school, or normal activities for more than one day per cycle, regularly.
- Pain during or after sexual intercourse (dyspareunia).
- Pain during bowel movements or urination, particularly at certain points of your cycle.
- Cyclical pain in unusual places shoulder, diaphragm, chest that worsens around your period.
- Pain that wakes you from sleep.

Bleeding

- Bleeding that soaks through a pad or tampon every hour for more than two consecutive hours.

- Passing blood clots larger than a ten-pence coin.

- Bleeding between periods.

- Bleeding after sex.

- Periods lasting longer than seven days.

- Post-menopausal bleeding (any bleeding after 12 months of no periods).

Fertility

- Trying to conceive for more than 12 months without success (6 months if aged 35 or older).

Other

- Severe fatigue with heavy bleeding possible anaemia requiring iron studies.

- A palpable lump or swelling in the abdomen.

- Significant weight loss alongside gynaecological symptoms.

- Pain or symptoms that are getting worse over time, not stable.

If you have any of these symptoms and have not been investigated, please return to your GP and request a referral. The phrase "red flag symptoms requiring investigation under NICE guidelines" is one that most GPs will take seriously.

Appendix D: NHS Specialist Endometriosis Centres

The British Society for Gynaecological Endoscopy (BSGE) accredits specialist endometriosis centres across the United Kingdom. These are hospitals with multidisciplinary teams including endometriosis surgeons, colorectal surgeons, urologists, pain specialists, and fertility consultants. If your endometriosis involves bowel, bladder, or other organs beyond the uterus, NICE guidelines recommend that you be referred to an accredited centre.

You are entitled to request referral to any BSGE-accredited centre in England, not only the one nearest to you. Many women travel for treatment. NHS Choice allows this.

The current list of accredited centres can be found at the BSGE website: bsge.org.uk/endometriosis-centres. Because the list is updated periodically, I have not reproduced it here to avoid the book becoming outdated. As of the time of writing, centres exist in most major English cities, including London (multiple), Birmingham, Manchester, Leeds, Liverpool, Newcastle, Bristol, Oxford, Cambridge, Sheffield, Nottingham, Southampton, Plymouth and others. Scotland, Wales, and Northern Ireland have their own specialist provision.

If your GP is unsure how to make a referral to an accredited centre, the phrase to use is: "I'd like to be referred to a BSGE-accredited endometriosis centre for multidisciplinary assessment." This is a formal referral pathway that exists in NHS commissioning documentation.

Appendix E: Resources and Advocacy Organisations

Endometriosis UK

National charity for endometriosis. Helpline, support groups, information, campaigns.

Helpline: 0808 808 2227 (Monday to Friday) | endometriosis-uk.org

Wellbeing of Women

UK charity funding research into women's reproductive and gynaecological health.

wellbeingofwomen.org.uk

Cysters

Charity supporting women from Black, Asian and ethnically diverse backgrounds with reproductive and mental health conditions.

cysters.org

The Adeno Gang

UK-based advocacy and support network for women with adenomyosis.

theadenogang.com

The Fibroid Network

UK support and information network for women with uterine fibroids, with particular focus on the disproportionate impact on Black women.

Black Womxn's Health

An advocacy and education organisation focused on health outcomes for Black women in the UK.

Five X More

Campaign to improve Black maternal health outcomes in the UK. Five action points for Black women, plus healthcare professional training.

fivexmore.com

Jamii

Supporting health and well-being for Black communities in the UK.

Foundation for Women's Health

Funds research into fibroids and other women's health conditions. Partnered with Lupita Nyong'o on the Uterine Fibroid Grant.

foundationforwomenshealth.org

Crisis support

Samaritans: 116 123 (free, 24 hours) | samaritans.org

NHS 111: for urgent non-emergency medical advice

Women's Aid: 0808 2000 247 (24-hour domestic abuse helpline)

The Lighthouse (Camden): services for children and young people who have experienced sexual abuse

Policy and government resources

The Renewed Women's Health Strategy for England (April 2026): available at gov.uk/official-documents

Hansard record of the 5 March 2026 Commons debate on Women's Health Strategy: Endometriosis and Fibroids: available at Hansard.parliament.uk

NICE Guideline NG73: Endometriosis (updated 2024): nice.org.uk/guidance/ng73

Acknowledgements

There is no such thing as a book written alone, and this one is less than most.

A book like this gets built out of the lives of the people who trusted it to hold the weight of what they had survived. So I want to begin, as I began in the Preface, with the women.

To every woman who sat with me, sometimes for hours, and told me, often for the first time out loud, what her body had been doing and what her doctors had not: thank you. You know who you are. Some of you are in these pages under your own names, and some of you are woven through the background of the argument, your experience part of the scaffolding, even where you did not want your name on it. Both are gifts. I have tried to be worthy of them.

To Jen Moore, who has spent more years campaigning on this than most politicians have spent in office, and whose line "we're just not believing women" is the centre of gravity of this book: thank you for the time, for the candour, and for the way you have refused, for more than two decades, to let the silence win.

To Hayley, to Sarah Beaton, to Natalie, to Etta, to Sophia and to the women whose names I have not been able to print here, at their request or for their protection. Your stories are not illustrations. They are the argument.

To Lupita Nyong'o: I do not know you personally, and likely never will, but I want to say here, in print, that the choice you made to sit in front of a television camera in February 2026 and speak plainly about seventy-seven fibroids and a ticking bomb and nobody helping that choice has rippled into the lives of more women than you will ever meet. There are women in this country who picked up the phone to their GP because you sat down with a morning show. Thank you for the cost of doing it in public.

※ ※ ※

To the British advocates and founders who have been holding the line in this country long before it became fashionable: thank you.

To Emma Cox and the team at Endometriosis UK, whose data has saved this book from a dozen errors and whose work has kept a generation of British women from thinking they were mad. To Neelam Heera-Shergill and the community at Cysters, whose refusal to let South Asian and Black women be treated as footnotes in this crisis has shaped how I wrote Part Four and shaped how I think. To Tanya Simon-Hall and the Adeno Gang, to the Fibroid Network, to Wellbeing of Women, to Black Womxn's Health, to Five X More, to Jamii, to every group chat and closed Facebook forum where women have been doing, without pay or thanks, the work the NHS should have been doing instead. You kept each other alive while the system decided whether you were interesting.

To the clinicians inside the NHS who have been quietly mutinous in the service of their patients: you know who you are, and why I cannot name all of you. Thank you for the referrals you fought for when the commissioning pathway said no. Thank you for the five minutes past the end of the appointment that you gave when the computer was flashing. Some of you are the reason women in this book are still here.

To Dr Itunu Johnson-Sogbetun, who, as a Black British GP, has been willing to say out loud what others will only whisper: that the stereotype of "normal for African women" is still alive in the consultation room, and that it is killing people. Thank you for the courage of that.

※ ※ ※

This book owes an enormous debt to the researchers and the research, and to the colleagues who trained me to read a paper properly and who have moved the science of women's health forward against a tide of underfunding and indifference.

To the Mary Seacole Awards, Health Education England, the Royal College of Midwives, the Royal College of Nursing, Unison and Unite, who made the original research possible and have continued to make space for Black women's voices in British healthcare when other institutions have not. To the Queen's Nursing Institute and the community of Queen's Nurses, who have taught me what it looks like to be in practice for decades and still angry on behalf of patients. To my colleagues at Middlesex University, where much of the thinking behind this book was born.

To the American Pregnancy Association and the global network of clinicians and researchers who have held open, across continents, the argument that women's bodies are worthy of investment. To the Foundation for Women's Health, currently funding the kind of fibroid research the NHS still has not chosen to. To the All-Party Parliamentary Group on Endometriosis, and to the MPs you know who you are who have been willing to say the word "scandal" inside the chamber rather than only outside it.

※ ※ ※

To the team at Vina, who have built, alongside me, the platform this book describes and who understand all of them that the book and the platform answer the same question. Thank you for making space for me to write, for cheering when chapters were done, and for holding the work while my attention was inside a manuscript. You are the quiet engine of this.

To my literary agent, who believed in a clinician's book with a fight in it before the market had proven there was one. To my editor, who knew when to push and when to leave a sentence alone, and who has made this a better book in every conversation. To the copy-editor who saved me from at least a dozen errors I would have carried to print. To the designer whose cover has already done some of the work the book has to do, and to the publicity team who believe, as I do, that silence is the one outcome we cannot afford.

To my previous readers, those who came to A Sister's Dream and Reframing Risk, Redesigning Care for staying with me across the arc of this work, and for writing to me, over the years, about the daughters and sisters and wives in your own lives who needed a book that did not yet exist. This is that book. Thank you for asking for it long enough that I had to write it.

※ ※ ※

To my family. To Parents in Zimbabwe who let me leave to build a life in which their daughter could grow up believing that her voice would be listened to, and who taught me sometimes by example, sometimes by argument that dignity is not granted by institutions, it is claimed in front of them.

To my brothers and sisters, who believe in me more consistently than I deserve. To the ladies of the family, the aunties, the cousins, the grandmothers, whose narratives of menstruation, suffering, midwives, and mothers inform every page of this book, whether I make it explicit or not. Thank you for the legacy.

To those who have suffered through me being partially present for long periods of writing, but who don't hold it against me. You know who you are. I promise to repay the favour someday, perhaps with another book.

※ ※ ※

Finally, to the reader.

If you are a woman who found herself in this situation, where she feels like something is going wrong and no one will believe her, and has turned to this book for help, I want you to know that you were at the forefront of my mind while writing this at all times. I imagine you holding this book in the bathtub at eleven PM, or sitting on the train reading this with a highlighter in your hand. I wanted to create this book, which could sit alongside you in these moments, affirming that you are right, that you are not alone, and that you don't have to keep it all bottled up inside anymore.

If you are a clinician, or a medical student, or a researcher, or a policy-maker, or someone in a position to change how any of this works, I want you to know I have thought about you, too. With, in many cases, more patience than I feel. The women in this book need you. I have tried to make the argument in a way that you can hear it.

If you are a partner, a parent, a friend, a colleague who has watched someone you love go through this and not known what to do, I hope this book gives you a language for it, and a reason to believe her the next time she tells you she is not well.

I am grateful that you are here. Books, at their best, are a form of company. This one is yours.

To every woman who was told she was making a fuss about nothing this was nothing. It was always the beginning of something.

Sarah Chitongo

References

All references are in Harvard style. Web sources were accessed during the research and writing of this book, between August 2025 and April 2026. Where URLs were included in the source material, these have been retained.

Primary government and policy sources

Department of Health and Social Care (DHSC) (2026) The Renewed Women's Health Strategy for England. London: HMSO. CP 1558. ISBN 978-1-5286-6262-8. Available at: www.gov.uk/official-documents.

Department of Health and Social Care (DHSC) (2022) Women's Health Strategy for England. London: HMSO.

Hansard (2026) 'Women's Health Strategy: Endometriosis and Fibroids', House of Commons debate, 5 March 2026, Volume 745.

NHS England (2026) Consultant-led Referral to Treatment Waiting Times Data 2025–26, January 2026. Incomplete Pathways Commissioner data file, National data table. Available at: england.nhs.uk.

Scottish Government (2026) Women's Health Plan Phase Two. Edinburgh: Scottish Government.

Welsh Government (2026) Women's Health Hubs Implementation Plan. Cardiff: Welsh Government.

National Institute for Health and Care Excellence (NICE) (2024) Endometriosis: diagnosis and management. NICE Guideline NG73, updated 2024. London: NICE. Available at: nice.org.uk/guidance/ng73.

Women and Equalities Committee (2024) Women's reproductive health conditions. House of Commons. Available at: parliament.uk.

Charity surveys and reports

Endometriosis UK (2024). The state of endometriosis care in the UK: A roadmap for driving down diagnosis times and improving access to care. London: Endometriosis UK.

Royal College of Obstetricians and Gynaecologists (RCOG) (2024) Waiting for a Way Forward: RCOG Gynaecology Waiting Times Tracker Report. London: RCOG.

Royal College of Obstetricians and Gynaecologists (RCOG) (2026) New Year: Still waiting for a way forward. London: RCOG.

Wellbeing of Women (2025). Just a Period: Calling Time on Heavy and Painful Periods. London: Wellbeing of Women.

Nurofen (2024). See My Pain: Gender Pain Gap Index Report. London: Reckitt.

Patients Association (2024) Prescription for Outpatients: A patient-centred approach to the redesign of outpatient services. Harrow: Patients Association.

Healthwatch Berkshire (2023) Women's Health Report: Findings from conversations with 580 women. Newbury: Healthwatch Berkshire.

British Pregnancy Advisory Service (2024). Contraception Re-Imagined: The Unfinished Revolution. London: BPAS.

MBRRACE-UK (2024) Saving Lives, Improving Mothers' Care 2024. Oxford: National Perinatal Epidemiology Unit.

Peer-reviewed research and academic sources

Bougie, O., Yap, M.I., Sikora, L., Flaxman, T. and Singh, S. (2019) 'Influence of race/ethnicity on prevalence and presentation of endometriosis: a systematic review and meta-analysis', BJOG: An International Journal of Obstetrics and Gynaecology, 126(9), pp. 1104–1115.

Buttram, V.C. Jr (1979) 'Endometriosis: its contemporary management', Fertility and Sterility, 31(2), pp. 117–123.

Chapron, C., Marcellin, L., Borghese, B. and Santulli, P. (2019) 'Rethinking mechanisms, diagnosis and management of endometriosis', Nature Reviews Endocrinology, 15(11), pp. 666–682.

Chatman, D.L. (1976) 'Endometriosis and the Black woman', American Journal of Obstetrics and Gynaecology, 125(7), pp. 987–989.

Chen, L.C., Hsu, J.W., Huang, K.L., Bai, Y.M., Su, T.P., Li, C.T., Yang, A.C., Chang, W.H., Chen, T.J., Tsai, S.J. and Chen, M.H. (2016) 'Risk of developing major depression and anxiety disorders among women with endometriosis', Journal of Affective Disorders, 190, pp. 282–285.

Chitongo, S., Pezaro, S., Fyle, J., Suthers, F. and Allan, H. (2022) 'Midwives' insights in relation to the common barriers in providing effective perinatal care to women from ethnic minority groups with 'high risk' pregnancies', Women and Birth, 35(2), pp. 152–159.

Criado Perez, C. (2019). Invisible Women: Exposing Data Bias in a World Designed for Men. London: Chatto & Windus.

Guzikevits, M., Gordon-Hecker, T., Rekhtman, D., Salameh, S., Gozal, D., Gileles-Hillel, A., Perry, A. and Chan, J. (2024) 'Sex bias in pain management decisions', Proceedings of the National Academy of Sciences of the United States of America, 121(33), e2401331121.

Huang, C.N., Stafford, M., Ayadi, F. and Briggs, A. (2023) 'General practitioners' views and experiences of menopause care: a qualitative interview study', British Journal of General Practice, 73(733), e675–e683.

Irving, G., Neves, A.L., Dambha-Miller, H., Oishi, A., Tagashira, H., Verho, A. and Holden, J. (2017) 'International variations in primary care physician consultation time: a systematic review of 67 countries', BMJ Open, 7(10), e017902.

Johnson-Sogbetun, I. (2024) 'What my Black patients don't say, and what I've learned to ask', essay published in clinical commentary series, accessed January 2026.

Katon, J.G., Plowden, T.C. and Marsh, E.E. (2023) 'Racial disparities in uterine fibroids and endometriosis: a systematic review and application of social, structural, and political context', Fertility and Sterility, 119(3), pp. 355–363.

Luo, J., Woodward, M., Ferreira, M.L. and Harris, K. (2026) 'Sex differences in the experience of pain in the UK Biobank cohort study', British Journal of Pain, 22, 20494637261418196.

Malory, B. (2023) 'The medical gaze and the communication of women's pain', in Communication, Medicine, Ethics. London: University College London.

McEwen, B.S. (2017) 'Neurobiological and systemic effects of chronic stress', Chronic Stress, 1, 2470547017692328.

Moseley, G.L. and Butler, D.S. (2015) 'Fifteen years of explaining pain: the past, present, and future', The Journal of Pain, 16(9), pp. 807–813.

Norman, A. (2018). Ask Me About My Uterus: A Quest to Make Doctors Believe in Women's Pain. New York: Nation Books.

Okoth, K., Chandan, J.S., Marshall, T., Thangaratinam, S., Thomas, G.N., Nirantharakumar, K. and Adderley, N.J. (2021) 'Association between the reproductive health of young women and cardiovascular disease in later life: umbrella review', BMJ, 371, m3502.

Ott, J., Fischer, E.M., Promberger, R., Kaufmann, U. and Egarter, C. (2012) 'Dietary habits of women with endometriosis', Reproductive BioMedicine Online, 25(6), pp. 559–565.

Palmer, M.J., Wellings, K., Graham, C. et al. (2025) 'Reproductive morbidity and associations with sociodemographic factors: findings from the Reproductive Health Survey for England', BJOG: An International Journal of Obstetrics and Gynaecology, 132(13), pp. 1782–1794.

Parazzini, F., Viganò, P., Candiani, M. and Fedele, L. (2013) 'Diet and endometriosis risk: a literature review', Reproductive BioMedicine Online, 26(4), pp. 323–336.

Perro, D., Hamilton, R., Joyce, K. and Mokoena, L. (2024) 'Unequal menstrual health: tackling the menstrual experiences of Black women in the UK', BMJ, 384, e075932.

Stewart, E.A., Cookson, C.L., Gandolfo, R.A. and Schulze-Rath, R. (2017) 'Epidemiology of uterine fibroids: a systematic review', BJOG: An International Journal of Obstetrics and Gynaecology, 124(10), pp. 1501–1512.

Tang, K. (2024). It's Not Hysteria: Everything You Need to Know About Your Reproductive Health (but Were Never Told). New York: Flatiron Books.

van Barneveld, E., Manders, J., van Osch, F.H.M., van Poll, M., Visser, L., van Hanegem, N., Lim, A.C., Bongers, M.Y. and Leue, C. (2022) 'Depression, anxiety, and correlating factors in endometriosis: a systematic review and meta-analysis', Journal of Women's Health, 31(2), pp. 219–230.

Journalism and media sources

BBC News (2025) 'Endometriosis: "I paid £10,000 for treatment after 12-year wait"', BBC News, accessed 2025.

Complex (2026) 'Lupita Nyong'o Opens Up About Living With "Over 50" Fibroids', Complex, 26 February 2026.

McKirdy, E. (2025) 'Scotland's gynaecology waiting list: the women waiting three years for care', published investigation, accessed 2025.

Refinery29 UK (2025) 'It Took Years To Be Heard: 4 Black Women On Their Struggle To Get An Endometriosis Diagnosis', Refinery29, March 2025.

STV News (2025) 'Scots woman Sarah Beaton discovers uterine cancer after paying £15,000 for private scan', STV News, February 2025.

TODAY (2026) 'Lupita Nyong'o Says Fibroids Have Returned:

EXCLUSIVE', NBC TODAY Show, 25 February 2026.

Nyong'o, L. (2024). Instagram posts on fibroids and Fibroid Awareness Month. July 2024. Available at: instagram.com/lupitanyongo.

Ethnicity, inequality, and organisational sources

NHS Race and Health Observatory (2024) Submission to Women and Equalities Select Committee Inquiry on Women's Reproductive Health. London: NHS Race and Health Observatory.

NHS England (2024) Adult Psychiatric Morbidity Survey 2023/4: Survey of Mental Health and Wellbeing, England. London: NHS Digital.

Office for National Statistics (ONS) (2025). The impact of an endometriosis diagnosis on monthly employee pay and employee status, England: April 2016 to December 2022. Newport: ONS.

Endometriosis Foundation of America (2025). Endometriosis Resource Portal for People of Colour, accessed 2025.

A note on citations in the text

Throughout this book, where I cite a source by name (for example, "DHSC, 2026" or "Endometriosis UK, 2024"), the full reference appears in this list. Where a quote from a named woman appears in published journalism, the journalism source is cited both at the point of quotation and in this list. Where a woman's story has been shared with me in confidence, her name has been changed, and this is flagged in the text. Nothing in this book is invented.

Any errors in citation, attribution, or fact that have survived into the published edition are mine, and I will correct them in future editions. Readers who identify errors are warmly invited to contact me via my publisher.

Made in the USA
Monee, IL
03 November 2026

67382321R00095